CW00494973

NOT THE ONLY ONE

Rachel Mason

Copyright © 2020 Rachel Marie Mason

All rights reserved

This book or any portion thereof may not be reproduced or used in any manner whatsoever without the express written permission of the author except for the use of brief quotations in a book review.

ISBN: 9798561703157

Cover design by: Emma Timms and Luke Pajak
Library of Congress Control Number: 2018675309
Printed in the United Kingdom

www.rachelmasonmusic.com
www.lyricallight.co.uk

DISCLAIMER

Although this publication is designed to provide accurate information in regard to the subject matter covered, the publisher and the author assume no responsibility for errors, inaccuracies, omissions, or any other inconsistencies herein.
This publication is meant as a source of valuable information for the reader, however it is not meant as a replacement for direct expert assistance. If such level of assistance is required, the services of a competent professional should be sought.

Although the publisher and the author have made every effort to ensure that the information in this book was correct at press time and while this publication is designed to provide accurate information in regard to the subject matter covered, the publisher and the author assume no responsibility for errors, inaccuracies, omissions, or any other inconsistencies herein and hereby disclaim any liability to any party for any loss, damage, or disruption caused by errors or omissions, whether such errors or omissions result from negligence, accident, or any other cause.

This is a work of nonfiction. No names have been changed (unless requested by the contributer), no characters invented, no events fabricated. Permission has been given by all contributers to use their stories and poems in this book.

For my three favourite people in the entire world, Tom, Layla and Elias.

FOREWORD

"You're not the only one"
I promise......

There are millions of fellow mums and dads around the world, questioning the darkness they feel shrouded in. Doubting if they are ever going to be that "perfect" parent. Feeling like they are failing at the one thing that was supposed to come naturally, and fearful that amongst the sea of incredible parents, cracking parenting every day, they are the only ones drowning......

Myself, the wonderful author of this book Rachel, and all the incredibly courageous men and women she has brought together over the following pages are here to reassure you that "No, you're NOT the ONLY one"
We are all here with you.

All of us are at different stages of our experiences battling the challenges our minds can throw at us after having a baby. All of us with our own individual and incredibly personal battles. But, all of us very much a part of the army of men and women around the world currently suffering, living with and survivors of a maternal mental health illness.

One of my biggest fears when I was suffering with my maternal mental health was that this was me now. That the old me had been lost forever and that the shell of a person I'd become, who was shrouded in fear and darkness, was who I was; was who I was going to be forever more.

I could not see a way out or a way forward and despite the well intentions of loved ones telling me everything was going to be okay, I simply did not believe them. They had not been through what I was going through. They did not have experience of a maternal mental health illness, so how did they know that I was going to be ok?

If I could have spoken to or read stories of women who had been through what I was going through, who had survived
it and come through to the other side, it would have been life changing for me. It would have given me hope. It would have given me strength to fight.

When I met Rachel in 2019 and learnt about the incredible work she does supporting mums with their maternal mental health through her Lyrical Light songwriting project I was completely blown away. Here was a fellow mum who had experienced the darkness of a maternal mental health illness and was now using her experiences in such a creative way to provide some light for fellow mums. It is a beautiful and empowering project and one that has helped so many men and women. And I know this beautiful book will go on to do the same.

This amazing book and the parents who have shared their

hearts and words are your reminder that you are not alone, that there is hope. They are your reminder to keep fighting no matter how dark the days get.

Do not give up on yourself.
With the right amount of love, support and care you will come through how you are feeling right now.

Please read this book and know that there is life after a maternal mental health illness and it is one worth fighting for!

Sending you lots of love and support,
Liv x

Liv Siegl is the best selling author of "Bonkers – A Real Mum's Incredibly Honest Tales of
Motherhood, Mayhem and Mental Health" (Harper Collins 2018), Expert Advisor on Global
Mental Health for the World Health Organisation and founder of The Letters of Light Project
– A global peer support project supporting women with their maternal mental health
around the world by sending handwritten letters of support from women with lived
experience of maternal mental health to women currently struggling.
www.lettersoflightproject.com

PREFACE

The Creation of Lyrical Light

During this book you will see some song lyrics. These were written at Lyrical Light songwriting workshops with mums and dads who were struggling with their mental health.

Here's the story of how Lyrical Light was created.

"My face wears a smile but my heart's full of tears"

That's a line I wrote for the song for an amazing group of women who attend a PANDAS Postnatal Depression Support Group. I visited them in July 2019 to run a songwriting workshop for them and was overwhelmed by their openness and kindness. They treated me as one of their own and made me feel surer than ever that being diagnosed with postnatal depression was not the end of the story, which was a massive comfort to me...

You see, I was also diagnosed with postnatal depression in December 2018 a year and a half after having our first child. I had given birth to our daughter in April 2017 and had silently suffered postnatal depression and psychosis but was too ashamed to tell anyone due to the stigma surrounding it. I painted on a smile and pretended to all the world that everything was fine, even shooting a television show for Sky One, recording an album and making a music video during this time but it felt like a shadow had been cast over my heart and nothing would lift it.

It was only after giving birth to our son in October 2018 and began to feel the same darkness and desperation that I finally reached out for help. With counselling, medication and the boundless love and support from my family and friends I now feel back to my old self again, most days.

I began to research postnatal depression while up at 3 am feeding the baby and realised not only how common it is but that there is so much support out there for those suffering.

I felt inspired to do something to help others so had the idea to set up Lyrical Light, a songwriting workshop for people with pre and postnatal depression. Since then I've been honoured to win Freelancer of the Year so have used some of the generous prize money to set up the business. I've been working with charities including PANDAS Foundation and Mother For Mothers, and companies such as PND And Me, Mothering Mental Health And Me, The Guilty Mothers Club, Mental Health Mates, The Postnatal Project and hospitals including Southmead and NHS Mother and Baby Units.

In 2019 Lyrical Light was awarded a Women In Business Award by Jacqueline Gold CBE.

Admitting I was struggling with postnatal depression has changed my life. I'm more open and willing to talk about the difficult times I've had. I still have some bad days but they are far fewer and I know they will pass. But best of all my admission has also drawn me into a loving and accepting community of amazing mums who also struggle with pre and postnatal depression. So many of these incredible women have told me that the very fact of knowing we are not alone has made it easier to get through the dark days.

Upon adding the finishing touches to the song for the mums at the PANDAS Postnatal Depression Support Group I wrote these lines that I now truly believe:

"The dark and despair seems to fade when you are there, For we are a light to illuminate the night."

Love Rachel x

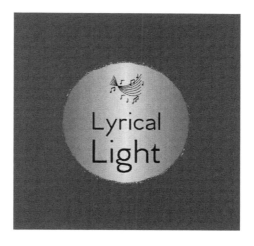

INTRODUCTION

What if I told you that you weren't the only one to feel depressed, angry, tearful and a million other things after having a baby?

I know because I'm one of the 1 in 7 women and 1 in 10 men who suffered with postnatal depression after the births of their children.

I'm a part of the statistic but that didn't make me feel any less alone. I didn't know anyone else I could talk to about my experiences as sadly postnatal depresison is still something not widely discussed. I felt isolated, left on my own little island adrift from the rest of the world.

One night when my daughter was 6 months old I couldn't sleep. I began searching through social media for anyone who spoke about their experiences with their mental health after having children. To my relief and surprise there were so many of them! I started to contact these amazing mums and dads who had been diagnosed with postnatal depression and other mental health issues and they began to share their stories with me.

An idea formed in my sleepy , frazzled mummy-brain.

What if I collated these these stories and made them into a book?

What if people could read the stories behind the statistics and know that they're not alone in this?

A matter of hours later I was sketching the outline for this book in a top covered in vomit with a baby lying across my lap.

Those who know me will have witnessed many of my creative ideas come to life and know how determined I am to make something happen if I think it will help others.

So I wrote this book for you; the mum desperately holding on, the dad holding back the tears, the family and friends not knowing how to help. I want you to know that you are not the only one, that you are loved and that every single contributer to this book gave their stories just for you.

HOW TO USE THIS BOOK

This book has been designed for busy mums and dads who simply do not have time to sit down quietly and read an entire novel.

Please feel free to pick it up and read a poem, an affirmation, a story or a set of lyrics and then put it down again. You don't need to read it in chronological order for it to "make sense". Just dip in and dip out as you please.

The book has also been designed to be compact so you can pop it into your baby change bag before heading off to the park, soft play centre or somewhere else where you just might get 5 minutes peace to read.

I've been assured it also fits nicely into a bathroom cupboard. I know that seems an odd thing to tell you but it's on the off-chance that you, like my friend, reads it when going to the toilet as that's the only time she gets a couple of minutes away from her toddlers!

CONTENTS

A LETTER OF LIGHT FOR YOU, DEAR READER

Dear Fellow parent,
I am writing this Letter of Light to let you know how incredible you are and what a fantastic job you are doing. I know you probably don't believe it right now and are feeling overwhelmed, but it is SO important to hold onto the fact that you can get through this.

I was once where you are now, feeling lost and undeserving of any sort of happiness. I felt cloaked in darkness and at my lowest of times felt that this was how my life was going to be forever. If you are feeling like this, I am here to tell you that this darkness will not last forever, with the right support you will come through this and you will be well again.

Please remember that how you are feeling is not your fault. You have done nothing to deserve how you are feeling right now. A maternal mental health illness does not discriminate, and it does not mean you have failed or are not a strong person. In fact, it means quite the opposite. The fact that you are battling this darkness every day means you are one of the bravest and strongest people out there.

I know we have never metbut I know what courage that takes, and I want to let you know how incredibly proud myself and all the other mums involved in The Letters of Light Project are of you.

We are all cheering you on and want you to know that you on not on your own! You have us all on your side, believing in you and sending you so much love and support.

On your darkest of days please read this Letter of Light as a reminder of how far you have come and to reassure yourself that there is life after a maternal mental health illness.

Most importantly never lose sight of how incredible you are and that you deserve the right to enjoy parenthood!

Sending you so much love and light,
Liv – A mum who cares xxxx
(Founder of The Letters of Light Project)

PERINATAL MENTAL ILLNESSES CHART

Estimated numbers of women affected by perinatal mental illnesses in England each year

1,380 Postpartum psychosis

Postpartum psychosis is a severe mental illness that typically affects women in the weeks after giving birth, and causes symptoms such as confusion, delusions, paranoia and hallucinations.
Rate: 2/1000 maternities

1,380 Chronic serious mental illness

Chronic serious mental illnesses are longstanding mental illnesses, such as schizophrenia or bipolar disorder, which may be more likely to develop, recur or deteriorate in the perinatal period.
Rate: 2/1000 maternities

20,640 Severe depressive illness

Severe depressive illness is the most serious form of depression, where symptoms are severe and persistent, and significantly impair a woman's ability to function normally.
Rate: 30/1000 maternities

20,640 Post traumatic stress disorder (PTSD)

PTSD is an anxiety disorder caused by very stressful, frightening or distressing events, which may be relived through intrusive, recurrent recollections, flashbacks and nightmares.
Rate: 30/1000 maternities

86,020 Mild to moderate depressive illness and anxiety states

Mild-moderate depressive illness includes symptoms such as persistent sadness, fatigue and a loss of interest and enjoyment in activities. It often co-occurs with anxiety, which may be experienced as distress, uncontrollable worries, panic or obsessive thoughts.
Rate: 100-150/1000 maternities

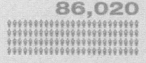

154,830 Adjustment disorders and distress

Adjustment disorders and distress occur when a woman is unable to adjust or cope with an event such as pregnancy, birth or becoming a parent. A woman with these conditions will exhibit a distress reaction that lasts longer, or is more excessive than would normally be expected, but does not significantly impair normal function.
Rate: 150-300/1000 maternities

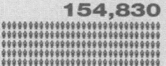

There may be some women who experience more than one of these conditions.
Source: Estimated using prevalence figures in guidance produced by the Joint Commissioning Panel for Mental Health in 2012 and ONS data on live births in England in 2011.

AWAKE

Like each phase of the moon
as it waxes and wanes
turning the tides that bind us to change
so when I pulse against this new me
like a heart inside it's chest
it is the moon, she reminds me
we will grow together

Holly Ruskin

HOLLY

The Perfect Bake

Before becoming a mother, I would follow recipes to the letter. I was exacting in my measurements; the stirring, beating and boiling.
My husband would gently chastise me as he liberally added ingredients that weren't on the list, in quantities that were nowhere near 'accurate'. Each time I would be sure of my triumph over his haphazard culinary efforts, yet somehow the end result – my finished dish – was always disappointing. It wouldn't look exactly like the picture or taste quite as good as I'd hoped. And still I persevered, slavishly trying to replicate what I'd found in the latest cookery book.

When my daughter was born, you could say I started out aproaching motherhood in the same way as my cooking.
A combination of an emergency c-section and subsequent birth trauma, mourning the loss of a natural birth, shock and extreme exhaustion was the perfect recipe for postnatal
depression.
I was anxious all the time. My heart raced. I was fearful of my daughter waking up and even more so of her being asleep. My house smelt different; my clothes fitted awkwardly on my body. I would sit beside my husband on the sofa weeping for how

much I missed him – and us. At my lowest ebb I said these words to him: "I don't want to leave her, but I want to leave". For almost a week, planning my escape was all that kept me calm.

My husband took me to the GP and within weeks I had a diagnosis and a prescription. In the midst of this physical and emotional upheaval, I reverted to what I knew. I clung to order and instruction like a life raft. I searched high and low for the perfect, easy to follow motherhood recipe.
Any time a well-meaning health visitor, midwife, friend or relative gave me a piece of advice, I followed it without question. I hired a lactation consultant and kept her plan next to me at all times, spending more time staring down at that dogeared piece of paper than at my beautiful girl as I nursed her. Our doula gave me a book – the third or fourth I'd read by this point – and I made us all miserable by obsessively following its schedule for days.

And yet, my baby remained her own little mystery. She came out a fully formed and unique person. Nothing was working, because I didn't need a recipe. She was already a perfect version of herself. A perfect bake.
Adrift in a sea of feeding and sleeping routines, I had simply lost my bearings. The waves of new motherhood crashed over me, leaving me feeling overwhelmed, frightened and alone.
All I'd wanted was a map I could follow that would bring me safely back to shore, to my old life and the me I was before.
I was lost.
Thankfully, that's not the end of this story. I wouldn't leave you here, though this might be where you are in your own mothering journey as you read this. And if so, here's what I want to say to you.

One night, when my daughter was around 6 months old, she

4

had woken for the sixth or seventh time since I'd nursed her to sleep. I was approaching an almost painful level of tired and had exhausted all the blogs, forums, books, podcasts and sleep experts. As I lay in bed watching car headlights sweep across the ceiling, it occurred to me that the only thing I hadn't tried was: nothing. I hadn't yet done absolutely nothing.

I knew that I was reaching another low point that I was afraid the tablets wouldn't be able to reach. The only person I really had left to help me was the one little person I had never thought to consult.

I slipped into my next snatched window of sleep with the determination to stop reading anything other than my daughter. The next morning I packed away every book I'd bought or been given. It was as though I had finally looked up from the page I was reading and saw her for the very first time. I don't follow recipes anymore. I cook with the joyful abandon of a maverick chef. There's not been a single meal I've made since cooking this way that I haven't enjoyed.

So, right here is where I'll leave you.

There will come a time when you'll return to yourself. You will run again. Laugh, listen to music, do a yoga class, read a book, take a bath, kiss your partner or cook a meal. It may be a slow return; a gentle approach back home to yourself. Or perhaps it will be more of a painful journey, each step deliberate and difficult. You could even find yourself in minutes, hours or mere days after becoming a mother. But however you get there, you will arrive back with you. For me it took one year. 365 days of taking the tablets, talking to other new parents, carving out small pockets of time for myself and soaking up the small moments of joy I finally found with my daughter. I started writing poetry and connected with a community of other mothers with whom I could share the light and the dark of motherhood.

5

Put down the books. Read your beautiful baby. Breathe. Breathe them in. Surround yourself with love and comfort. Trust your instincts. Your life is waiting for you on the other
side of your motherhood mountain. And when you get there, live it like you've never read a single recipe book in your life.

RISE

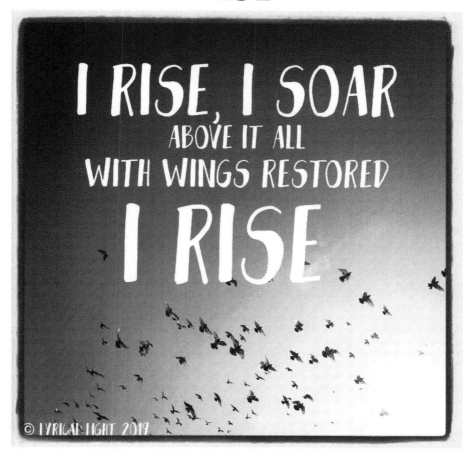

CHASM

Yours is a chasm of need I must fill
with nothing but myself to offer
never knowing all the while
if that will be enough

Holly Ruskin

VANESSA

A Mother Is Born Too

Having a baby for me was mentally a reverse experience of many women's stories.

I experienced pretty bad mental health issues from about the age of 15. At 17 I took an overdose and was admitted to hospital for 3 days. It was awful. The ward I was put in was full of strangely-behaved people. One woman pretended to be a nurse and came round to see me in the middle of the night. The next day a psychiatrist bullied me into answering her hard questions. "Why did I do it? Why?" My mum gave me a teddy. I didn't think I deserved it.

At 21 the problems grew beyond belief. I would be talking with friends and suddenly have a terrible buzzing in my head which meant I couldn't hear what anyone was saying. I was too scared to tell anyone but kept telling myself to see it through one more day.

During this time, I had an abnormal reaction to the idea of having a baby. I would anxiously wait for my period to arrive and then sigh with relief when it came, just before having cramping that was so bad I often took an (unpaid) day off work.

I've always felt I behaved differently from other women – not just about having a baby but about many matters, emotionally and aspirationally.

I wasn't sure having a baby was for me. But when I met my husband, he was Catholic and I had to make a promise in church not to obstruct the path for having children. I knew I had to honour it.

Part of me must have wanted a child but when I eventually got pregnant (which took some time), I couldn't be happy in the way I wanted to be. The questionnaire I was given by my midwife meant it came up and they sent me to a psychologist. I went twice, had to face two of them together and found the whole experience horrid. Then I contacted them to say I wasn't coming again and they wrote back suggesting I didn't like getting in touch with my feelings.

The truth was, I'd started hypnobirthing lessons and it was so wonderful that I felt the psychoanalysis was getting in the way.

Hypnobirthing taught me to be much calmer and not catastrophise a situation. So I really didn't need people prodding around in my past bringing up unhelpful memories.

However, I honestly didn't believe I felt anything about the baby. It was so strange having my family and friends be so pleased for me. I was numb to it all. I felt guilty as I knew how much some people longed for a baby. I didn't deserve one.

In addition to this, I had a very strong reaction to the idea of a c-section. I felt as though I could get through anything as long as I had a natural birth. But when my waters broke there was meconium and I was immediately sent to the central delivery unit, full of machines and numerous doctors.

Thankfully, I'd learnt in hypnobirthing I could say no to things. The hideous drip. The intense pressure by the doctors to have a caesarean. And somehow they found a way to get me through it.

At just after midnight my son was born and I was ecstatic. I'd made it through without surgery! And then I saw him: a tiny little face with a bow for a mouth and I thought,

"So that's what you look like".

I'd thought all babies looked the same.

Over the coming weeks, I couldn't have been more delighted. I loved being a mum, I honestly thought it was all going to be terrible. Part of me wonders if I'd made it so awful in my head that anything better was wonderful by comparison, but I know that's not true.

I also know, however, that things could have gone the other way. I was very lucky to love being a mum. But I could so easily have had a different experience.

I'd never pressure anyone to become a parent and I certainly wouldn't joke, "you'll love it when they're born!"
Anyone who says that doesn't know the terrifying depths a mind can go to.

SKINS

Some days I slip
between the skins of who I am now
and who I was then,
both of them chafing
not quite growing or shedding,
so though my love for you is in my bones
I miss the skin that held them in
the one I grew before I made you

Holly Ruskin

ILLUMINATE
THE NIGHT

My face wears a smile but my heart's full of tears
In the moments I'm left in the dark,
Over the months through all these cares
I see that life's faded my spark.
The colours are muted, their vibrancy gone
As I spiral down once again,
But I know that night will give way to the dawn
When you walk with me through the rain.
My hand in your hand

Your words in my heart
Shoulder to shoulder
United we'll start.
The dark and despair
seems to fade when you're there
For together we're a light
To illuminate the night.
Some days I'm happy, some days I'm numb
Some days a ghost drifting through,
But all my bad days don't make me a 'bad mum'
I'm stronger than I ever knew.
So try to live lightly, be kind to your mind
Be proud of who you have become,
The woman you are has been redefined

A brave mother who has overcome.
My hand in your hand
Your words in my heart
Shoulder to shoulder
United we'll start.
The dark and despair
seems to fade when you're there
For together we're a light
To illuminate the night.

Rachel Mason

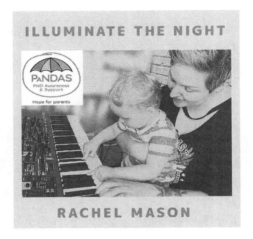

EMMA

Becoming Mum

We always planned to have two children, but our family of four came via a different route to the one we started out on.

My husband and I grew our lovely little family through adoption, with our little ones (siblings) being placed with us, their forever family, aged 3 and 4 years several years ago.

We were under no illusions that our lives were about to change in a huge way, with the arrival of two walking, talking, highly anxious and traumatised little children, but nothing can truly prepare you for parenthood, and this was no different in that respect. We were both excited and nervous about this significant life change for all of us.

Those early days with the children are a bit of a blur if I'm honest. I remember working really hard to build a relationship with my children, to anticipate their every need, be consistent, present and empathic, and be the best co-regulator I could as they were so easily, and understandably, regularly overwhelmed by their emotions. We weren't able to see close family and friends for a while as we'd been encouraged to spend quality time with the children without introducing other people into the mix. Introducing others was a slow and carefully planned out process. Everything was focused on helping the children feel safe in their forever family. I became obsessed with reading adoption forums and creating visuals to help the children get into a new routine.

Throughout all of this, I would experience repeated high levels of rejection. My husband got some of that but it was nowhere near the same level as for me, no matter how hard I tried, my kids seemed unable to even begin to accept me as a caring, loving mother and that really hurt.

I began to feel like an outsider in my own home as our children made me feel like they and my husband were in a little club I was not allowed to be part of. I know why this was the case (my kids were (understandably) operating from a place of fear, and had learned to respond in certain ways to adults around them in order to protect themselves), but when you're emotionally invested in trying to be the best parent you can and it's thrown back in your face no matter how hard you try, it is incredibly difficult not to take it personally. I shared my feelings with my husband but we were both trying to navigate a new intense dynamic together, so it wasn't easy for him either.

We both worked hard at presenting a united team front and I just kept going, not feeling like I had much choice but to push through and hope for chinks of progress, but increasingly feeling like a failure.

About 3 months after the children arrived, I started to feel particularly low and a shadow of my former self, almost resigned to things being this way forever. I felt we were living in an intense, and at times very dark bubble. Our children required huge amounts of containment, close supervision, extra reassurance and so much support with everything - the enormity of the responsibility for helping them to heal, while trying to bond as a parent, was heavy and there was no break from any of it.

We tried to do fun things with the children, but that would get sabotaged. The children couldn't cope with excitement or much outside of a very basic routine; it was just too overwhelming for them.

The levels of rejection I experienced, the emotions I absorbed while trying to help my little ones (secondary trauma is real), the exhaustion from trying to parent two hyper-vigilant young children and the high expectations I placed on myself to be the perfect therapeutic mum took their toll.

On top of all of this was the guilt - being a mum really didn't feel like I thought it would and I felt terrible about that. Everybody around us had been so excited for us to welcome children into our lives but I wanted to scream

'where's this joy everyone talks of, and this immediate rush of love?'.

Adoption is so often talked about in terms of 'happy ever after' in wider society, and that brings with it its own weight of expectation. Of course I know now that for us, real love was to come with time, and that is okay, but hindsight is a wonderful thing. I grieved the loss of the family I thought we would be while I kept going and hoped things would change.

A few weeks later, I went to an adoptive mum's support group, aware that not only was my state of mind not healthy for me, but this probably wasn't helping my kids feel safe either. I distinctly remember saying 'please someone tell me it gets better' as I sat down in the room, to which there was a long pause and someone piped up with

'mmmmm....I can't say it gets any easier but things change'.

I also remember considering turning around and walking straight back out again as that was not the answer I'd gone there for, but I stayed and listened to everyone's experiences all the same. I understood there and then that I was not alone in how I was feeling, but that I needed some external support.

The next day I phoned our social worker and asked to be referred to a specialist counsellor. Thankfully he was able to put me in touch with someone relatively quickly, and the sessions were funded as part of post-adoption support. Those 6 sessions were a godsend. Space and time to myself and the ear of someone who didn't judge, who had been there and done that (my counsellor was also an adoptive parent). They gently helped me realise that the way forward was to start with some more self-compassion as I'd increasingly been putting my own basic needs last and placing unrealistic expectations on myself.

Off the back of that, I started to find more opportunities to do things for 'me' and to prioritise my own needs without feeling selfish (though I'll be honest, the not feeling selfish bit is a work in progress...).

A short while after the counselling finished, I reconnected with music. Music had previously been a big part of my life (I'd literally crawled to the piano as a toddler, picking out simple tunes, and taught music in primary schools in my first employment), but I'd somehow drifted away from it over the years and realised how much I'd missed it. I found a fabulous vocal coach as I'd always wanted singing lessons when I was younger and never gotten around to it, despite singing in lots of choirs and at family parties for years. Singing is so therapeutic and a great way to relieve tension. I enjoy honing my skills along the way and I get a real sense of achievement
when I master a new vocal technique or explore different styles.

I also see my lesson time as a space for me, away from the day to day family-work juggle. I sang in a concert in front of my kids for the first time a couple of Christmas' ago, and they sat beaming with pride the whole way through (yes, I did get choked up!). My daughter finds so much joy in singing too,which is lovely.

So I guess looking back, it took some time, lots of introspection and some external help to work through that first year or so as a mum, but my kids (and husband!) now benefit from a mum who models self-compassion and has more energy and patience. Through finding a bit more of the old me again I got some sparkle back along the way. When I'm regulated, rested, and fulfilled my children naturally seem more able to cope as they inevitably pick up on my energy, and that allows us all to experience more joy within one anothers' company.

We have a strong bond - it's been hard work consistently building that, but of course our kids deserve nothing less - and we have very much settled into our 'normal' as a family which is still very routine-based and not without significant challenges but we are (for the most part) thriving, rather than just surviving. I now make a concerted effort to take account of my own needs within our family schedule (which also includes enough quality time with friends and wider family, and accepting help where it is offered).

The balance isn't always right, but I know when it's been off for just a bit too long and how important it is to reset it.

SURVIVAL GUIDE

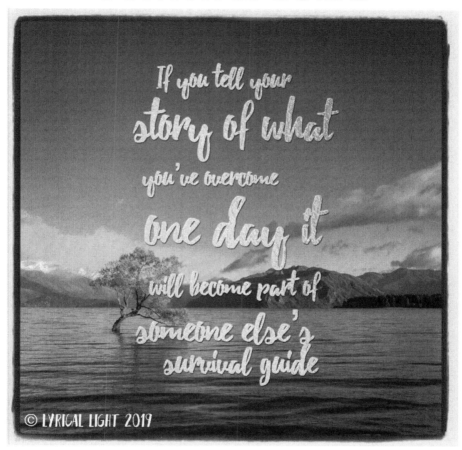

If you tell your story of what you've overcome one day it will become part of someone else' survival guide

© LYRICAL LIGHT 2019

HOMEGROWN

Skin within skin
bone over bone
my love for you is
homegrown

Holly Ruskin

MICHAEL

Every Tear Will Be Wiped Away

How on earth do I deal with this? I cannot do this? Why me?

I will never forget this one poignant Sunday morning; it was my turn to get up with our two kids to do their breakfast. I was standing in the kitchen making a cup of tea, stirring the tea bag. In that moment all I wanted to do was take my own life. I just could not take the depressive and suicidal thoughts anymore. I wanted to run away from this situation. It really felt like it would be so much easier if I were not here anymore. No parent should ever have to face the reality of witnessing their child die in their lifetime and this was something that could happen at any time for me.

Every morning I woke up thinking was my son gone. I just could not bear it anymore. All the great times, playing and laughing together, gone in an instant. It was too much to comprehend.

You never think it will ever happen to you but in an instant your world can so easily be turned upside down. It has been just over two years since being in that small hospital room. Yet is still feels like it was only yesterday when I had to walk down this cold endless corridor into an eerily quiet appointment room. As I waited with my wife for what seemed an age in this uncomfortable chair, having to watch couples come in and out, I wanted to be positive about this situation but I knew deep down that something was wrong.

Up to that point, life had been great, doing a job I absolutely love, married to an amazing wife and father to a beautiful daughter. However, in this small room I was listening intently to the words of the consultant tearing my world part as I sobbed my heart out. The consultant told us that our unborn son had a congenital heart defect. He was diagnosed with Tricuspid Atresia and Transposed Great Arteries, with two big holes in the Heart wall between the ventricle heart chambers.
The outlook was scary, bleak, and unknown.

Even though the consultant was giving us some hopeful words about future operations to make best his situation and give him a fighting chance of survival, I was an absolute mess. I foolishly thought it would be the other way around with myself being ok and my wife being upset, but it totally was not. She was my absolute rock and she took it so well, whereas I was all over the place. It felt like I was grieving for his death before he has even been born. As a father, I was totally inadequate to do anything about it, as if I ever could.

As time went on, I fell into that typical stereotype male thinking that I should be the strong one here and I bottled all my hurts, pains, and depression. My response was always 'I am fine' but it eventually got too much for me and I was at breaking point. I really could not tell you what made me make this decision, but I knew I had to go see a professional to get help. Fortunately, my wife had seen a therapist many years back and I felt like I could confide with him because there was already a connection and he knew our situation. I know this may not always be the case for many people but having a good relationship makes a massive difference to any counselling being effective.

It was one of the best decisions I ever made because he gave me a new perspective on life. He listened to everything I had to say and gave me permission to know it is ok not to be ok. It's ok to have those days where I don't feel great or cry it I need to. Most importantly he helped me to focus my thoughts on one or two good things that happen daily with my son. This really helped me to ignore my negative thoughts and see the wonderful blessing that he is.

I know that I cannot always stop my suicidal thoughts or thoughts of my son dying, but I can choose to enjoy the small moments like when he laughs his head off, or when he says funny words or gives me an unexpected hug. He literally makes me feel like this whole situation does not exist.
Presently, my son is between planned open-heart surgeries. Even though you can see glimpses of where his half heart is affecting him, overall, he is doing really well and developing brilliantly. I know the future is unknown and there may well be many difficult days to come.

What has really kept me going is my relationship with Jesus because I know that whatever happens to my son, whether he lives or dies, Jesus has secured his future, eternally and that gives me such hope that this difficult life will not overcome us as a family. My wife and I are going to make the most of every moment we have with him and are so thankful for the life he has.

MOTHER TO CHILD

Mother to child
A bond so strong
Carved in my heart
Like an angel's song.
Child to mother
You've set me free
Reached through the
dark
To rescue me.

© Lyrical Light 2019

AYMEE

A New Way Of Living

I wasn't diagnosed until I took my children in, to evaluate their mental health. My symptoms were always there, however, for as long as I can remember; quiet and in the background.

As I matured into adulthood they got loud. No longer content with their previous settings. Telling me things I couldn't control. Compelling me to take greater risks. Leaving me feeling raw, empty, and wishing for an off button to quiet my spinning brain.

I didn't know there was a name for what I was experiencing; that it could be defined and treated. I just believed I was crazy. Alone, different, and quietly suffering in my head.

After having children everything intensified. I felt such a crushing weight to life; an overwhelming and suffocating weight. How was I supposed to care for this new life when I was barely hanging on to my own? The days seemed to last forever, and the nights were filled with an uncontrollable mind that wouldn't quiet.

One child became two. As they grew I began to notice things. Some looked a little too familiar while others completely stumped me. Social problems outside the "norm" as early as 18 months. Tantrums that couldn't be soothed. An obsessive need to have things a certain way. And I saw for my children what I couldn't see for myself. They needed help. They needed support beyond my understanding and skill.

It was during a specific evaluation for my youngest that I finally felt understood. She was being screened for OCD as part of the testing process. I was given pages of questions to rate on a scale. With my daughter in mind, I began reading. Shortly after, I noticed a shift. I stopped thinking of her and saw the questions relating to me. Explaining things I could never admit out loud. Things I thought made me a monster. Things no one could ever know. Tears started streaming down my face. Questions became a blurry mess as emotions flooded me.

At each new appointment for my children, I was given the opportunity to evaluate what I saw in them and also in myself. By the time I saw a doctor, I had a pretty good idea of my diagnosis; a handful of labels that helped me understand myself in a way I never had before. The appointment went pretty much how I expected, having been through so many with my kids. I left with confirmation of what I had already found and a treatment plan.

I have always been an advocate for medication ever since my

oldest started at a young age and we saw the difference it could make. I knew the probability of having it recommended for my-self, and I was ready...or so I thought. When my doctor said one of the biggest supports for living a full life with OCD, was medication, I experienced a wave of emotions I wasn't expecting. I felt like a failure; like a problem that needed "fixing". What did it say about me, that I needed to be medicated to have a quiet brain? To have a brain that didn't tell me horrific things; a brain that didn't compromise my innate moral compass. It was very unexpected. I had never thought these things in relation to my daughters, but when it was my turn, it felt different.

Acceptance came with time; with therapy and the support of a husband who never looked at me differently after the diagnosis. A husband who knew I was the same person I had been before; who accepted fully, and listened to the things I was previously too scared to say out loud.

Through medication, therapy, self-care, and support, I have found a new way of living; one that has light and hope. One that can pull me up when I feel overwhelmed. I still don't fully understand my experience, or my children's. I still have dark days. I still have dark months with OCD controlling me. But the knowledge I have, the resources I've utilized, and the support I've found have given me the opportunity to succeed.

Two kids became three and as a family of five, we are constantly working toward a better future. We are constantly learning and growing as we navigate this world of mental health. And most importantly we are honoring our natural selves by supporting our weaknesses and growing in our strengths.

REFUGE

A slow untangling of myself from me,
an unravelling and undoing
of who I thought I'd be as a mother;
peeling back each layer
until I reach the hushed centre of my storm
finding my love for you there as a fixed point,
no moving with the seasons
the turn of a leaf or the setting sun
so it's here I seek my refuge
and the place I'll come to rest

Holly Ruskin

ASK FOR HELP

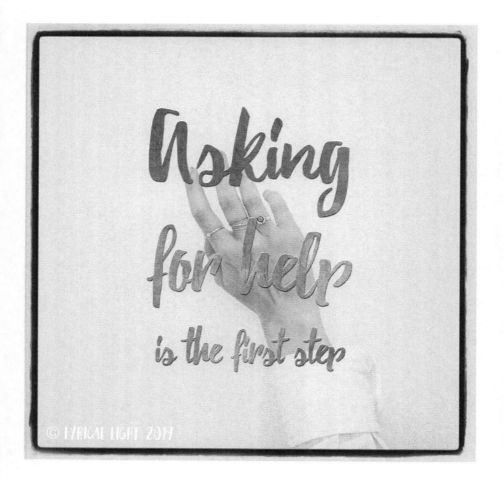

STEPHANIE

A New Way To Communicate

L ast year should have been a happy time giving birth to my second gorgeous little boy Reggie, but it was also the worst time of my life.

I have been suffering with postnatal depression since Reggie was 3 weeks old, my husband turned around to me one day and said about going to speak to my doctor about my emotions and low moods that had been going on.

I did go to the doctor and am now still having support from my doctor and my mental health nurse. It's scary to look back on all the bad days that I had and on the times I felt so low that I ended up self harming. When I was in those dark moments it felt like I wasn't in control of myself and it wasn't me that was doing those things.

I was then admitted to a mental health hospital in Winchester for mothers and babies when Reggie was just under 4 months old. It was the hardest thing I had ever had to do as I had to leave my eldest son Archie at home even though he was only three years old. However I knew that I needed to do this to become the best mum I could be for both my boys. All the staff were so friendly and it also helped being around other mums in the same situation and I began to feel that I wasn't alone being with other people going through this hard time too.

After about a month of being at the hospital and being involved in groups and also one to one meetings with my consultant and the nurses there, I thought I was ready to come home and to start my recovery process at home with my family, little did I know that I actually wasn't ready to come home.

A couple of weeks later I really hit rock bottom and I didn't want to carry on with my life. I felt so tired and lifeless and like shit all the time. Then came one weekend at the beginning of December. I don't really remember too much about it except that I just felt numb and that my head was like a black hole. I ended up taking an overdose of medication because I wanted all the pain and thoughts to stop and go away; I just wanted to fall asleep and not wake up.

When I woke up in hospital I could feel that someone was looking over me and telling me that I am strong and I can get through this, I just needed to believe in myself.

Then 2020 hit. It has been a tough year for everyone and it has most certainly been tough for those that suffer with mental illness. I am in the process of completing a 12 week course called Emotion Coping Skills with my mental health nurse and other mums that have also been having their own struggles. With speaking out, asking for help, being on the right medication and also having all the support around me I have become a much stronger person and I truly believe that anyone can get through this horrible illness. You just need to believe in yourself like everyone else believes in you.

I was never good at speaking to people about how I felt, so the one thing that made it easier for me was that if I was having a bad day then I would text my husband, even if he was in the same room as me. I would tell him how I was feeling and I would say that I am not ready to talk about it, so at least he knew how I felt, and that I was quite vulnerable to the things that were going on around me. He would then either give me a big cuddle or he would say
"Go and have a nice bath. Try and relax and do some mindful meditation" which again is another thing I have loved doing.

When someone at the start of my journey told me to try some meditation I thought how the hell is this going to work, but it is absolutely amazing and I love it. Most evenings before I go to bed I do some mindful meditation and it truly helps me relax. My body switches off and it also helps me get off to sleep with positive thoughts not negative. Sometimes I go into such a deep sleep that my husband then removes my head phones as I have fallen asleep in bed listening to my meditation.

Give anything a go if someone mentions an idea to try and help you. Some things work for people but also sometimes they don't. Everyone is different and by trying a few different things you will be able to find the things that best help you.

Always believe in yourself. Don't feel ashamed asking for help. This is my story and this is proof that anything is possible.
Keep believing, keep smiling.

TRAPPED

Wanting to leave
but not wanting to leave you,
trapped between your needs
and my need to be alone,
this conflict marking off
the darker days of mothering

Holly Ruskin

FILL YOUR CUP

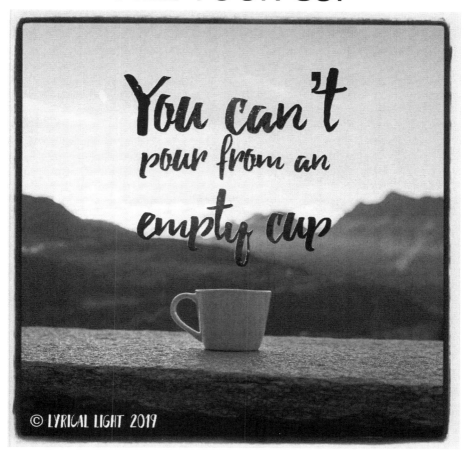

DANIEL

The Eye Of The Storm

I t was my partners and my first pregnancy and we were young. I was 18 at the time of the birth and my partner was 17.

The pregnancy was almost textbook with little complications other than our little one deciding not to come on time. We were excited as although she was not exactly planned we had spoken about the possibilities of having our own little family
so some might say she was a little surprise, but in a good way.

The labour started off very normal and my partner decided to opt for the epidural to help ease her pain but a few hours later we had concerned doctors, midwives and a very concerned nurse in the shape of my now mother-in-law as the baby was not moving downwards and her heartbeat was becoming irregular.

The doctor decided it best to rush to theatre and use the suction cap to help pull the baby out of the birth canal. As the dad I was gowned up and taken in to be by my partner's side which was very scary BUT it was not my job here to show worry or stress, instead it was my job to calm and comfort my partner.

After what seemed like forever the baby was born healthy and screaming and I took a sigh of relief after all this should have been it!? But not 10 minutes into parenthood and the feeling of the theatre room changed. What felt like the eye of the storm had passed over us and here we were right back in the storm. My partner had started to bleed out and was losing blood very fast as she was in the midst of a PPH (Post-partum haemorrhage). The midwife tried to reassure me but my history of hospitals and dealing with doctors from a young age due to my mum and dad's issues made me very aware that all was not right. I was quickly told to leave the room and to take my baby daughter with me.

The moment I saw my mother in law, Sue I felt as if I had let her down in looking after her daugher and I used my baby Ava as a means to try and take her mind off the situation as well as a way to get myself alone. I gave Ava to Sue to hold and told her what was happening. I was breaking down and yet found myself trying to hold it in for the sake of Sue and Ava but inside I had so many thoughts, the picture that was coming back to me was the big bag of Hannah's blood underneath Hannah and the thought that just like my mum, Hannah was not coming out alive.

This was cut short as Hannah was screaming for her mum and due to her being a nurse they let her in to be with Hannah. Finally I was alone with Ava and as I looked down at her I broke down.

I remember thinking I could not do this alone. I could not lose someone else this close to me. Pictures of my mum lying dead on the hospital bed would not leave my mind. I was alone with

Ava depending entirely on me and it felt too much. I needed someone to just take Ava so I could be alone completely.

I needed for it all to go away and be ok, but nothing came. I was on the verge of being a complete mess until a midwife came out to check on me as Hannah during all her medical issues had begged someone to check in on me as she knew I would be a mess. As soon as the midwife came I pulled it all back, she could tell I had been crying but chose to ignore it and instead tried to get my mind off things by getting me to dress Ava. This was not my job. Hannah wanted to do this but here I was doing it.

After what seemed like forever Hannah was wheeled out shaking violently due to the drugs that had been pumped into her and due to the loss of blood. They had fixed her and saved her! at that moment in time she was my hero and no words can describe the immense relief I felt just seeing her alive and awake in front of me!

Even though I have never felt as though I needed any help for what I went through that's not to say I didn't have any issues. For some time I found myself dreaming of being back in that theatre room and took a while to come to terms with what had happened.

Maybe getting help would have been a better solution than coping on my own but I felt that as though it wasn't me that had gone through the birth I shouldn't make a fuss. I felt like a fraud in a way but now I'm proud to say I can look back and feel ok to talk about this time in my life.

NIGHT

Nothing for it
in the dead of night
but to hold on

Holly Ruskin

CATHERINE

Never Alone

Given my history of depression and anxiety stemming from previous eating disorders and self-harm, I should have perhaps been more aware that I needed to take extra care of my mental health during my pregnancy.

I didn't comprehend how much my anxiety following a previous baby loss would spill over into the birth and postnatal period.

Despite a traumatic birth, Jake arrived safely into the world with a loud wail. Relief washed over me instantly but that was soon replaced with a feeling of numbness and shock. It was a surreal feeling to have a healthy living baby in my arms.

I felt overwhelmed, exhausted and disoriented.
I felt numb and cut-off from the situation in front of me. My mind was paralysed with fear as I held him. We were prompted to dress and place a nappy on him but I couldn't remember what to do and it terrified me. My mind was blank and I was panick-

ing. I wanted to turn and run.

I cried uncontrollably, huge great big racking sobs as I wondered what I had done. I honestly felt as though I had made the worst decision of my life. I couldn't shake the thought of wanting to leave and never come back.

Looking back now, I was a prime candidate for Postnatal Depression. I never noticed the subtle symptoms at first. I cried a little more and wrote it off as hormonal changes. I slept a little less; lying awake panicking about something happening to Jake, and I skipped a few meals due to the uneasiness I felt in the pit of my stomach about my new role.

As the days wore on, the anxiety that had been masked by shock returned with full force. Simple tasks such as leaving the house on time for an appointment or preparing a meal came with an unbearable weight to be executed perfectly.

I felt a wave of immense failure when I didn't achieve my own expectations of motherhood. My reality turned out to be so wildly different.

One day, I cried heavily as Jake bawled next to me on the sofa and I realised I couldn't hide it anymore. My new life was nothing how I had imagined, yet I felt very ashamed. What was I doing so wrong?

My partner called The Perinatal Team when I retreated to my bed under the weight of despondency and melancholy.

The consultant was so concerned with my behaviour which emanated in me being unable to be in the same room as Jake. When I expressed a desire to have him adopted she suggested an admission to a Mother and Baby Unit.

My mood was so low I thought my baby would be better off without me and I attempted to take my own life. What followed was 4 months of intensive support, extreme emotional turmoil, a relationship on its knees and several physical wounds, but we were discharged with a new lease of life and I threw myself into motherhood with an excitement I had never experienced before.

My recovery has had many peaks and troughs. One of the greatest empowerments was owning my own motherhood. I'd been fed this fairytale by society; a smooth and uplifting birth; a mother that exclusively breastfed, glowing in her new role, and a baby that slept beautifully which gave the time to represent an impeccable appearance and household. Once I realised I didn't need to seek validation from others or measure up to what a book said I blossomed in a way I never could have imagined. I'm finally the mum I'd always wanted to be and we're both happier as a result. I can ultimately shrug off comments from others when they tell me I'm doing it wrong. That no longer rips apart my confidence and you know what, that feels AMAZING.

The fact that my story has further opened up the conversation for maternal mental health and helped shine a light on postnatal mental illness is monumental. If it aids other mothers to feel unashamed in their emotions or guides them to spot the early warning signs of depression or psychosis, thus seeking the vital help they need then I can wholeheartedly say that publicly exposing my struggles has been a positive action.

I know that now I am completely recovered. Jake and I now have the most beautiful bond. I never thought this could be achieved when I was in the darkest depths of postnatal depression but here we are. I cherish every moment because once upon a time, it wasn't like this.

Baby loss and postnatal depression changes a mother forever but despite experiencing the ruthless, relentless and utterly dark side of motherhood, I feel I am a better person because of it. I have deeper empathy for others, endless compassion and a passion that runs though my veins to help other mothers. I never want anyone else to ever feel as isolated and despairing as I once did.

Recovery is possible. However bad you might be feeling right now please know that it won't be this way forever. Change is possible. Holding onto that spark of hope is essential in times of complete desperation, so please remember you are never EVER alone.

WEEDS

Shattered by your needs
those early weeks
they broke me
but through the cracks
light came seeping
and so like weeds
love grew

Holly Ruskin

QUIET THE STORM

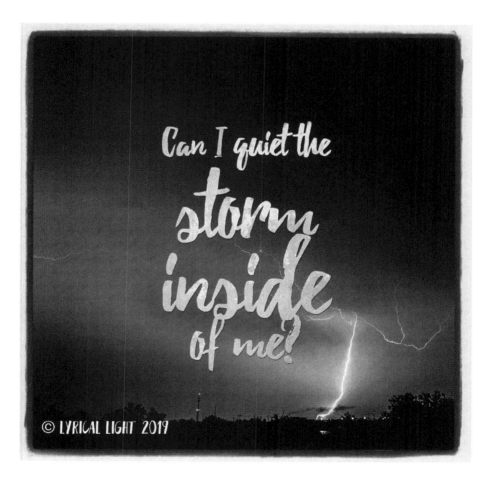

MARIA

Finding The Jigsaw Pieces

Almost a decade ago I suffered and recovered from Post-natal Illness (PNI). I have never been a wordsmith but I will endeavour to walk you through my PNI journey and if my tale sometimes seems messy, that might give you an insight into how it all felt. In fact during my illness writing a two-line text was often way beyond my ability. I am dyslexic and my ability to read and write was further impeded.

In truth I hid my illness from almost everyone close to me due to the stigma associated with maternal mental health, but also due to the fact that I could not understand what was wrong with me and why I was unable to be like all the other Mums out there. I felt tremendously guilty and ashamed of myself.

◆ ◆ ◆

William

Like many other women, my journey into motherhood was not straightforward. I had a number of early miscarriages before becoming pregnant with my first son.

I had a wonderful pregnancy with him, I felt happy and healthy, enjoyed every minute and excitedly planned a perfect home birth. At 11 days overdue I walked up a hill in the snow to the hospital for a wellbeing scan. Naively I did not take a hospital bag with me as I did not intend to stay to give birth. Later that day I was induced and after 19 hours William was born by forceps in theatre, a very different birth experience to the one I had hoped for. But he was here, I was happy and I fell immediately in love with him. He cried and was then rushed to NICU. 24 hours later he died in my arms.

The care and compassion my husband and I received in hospital following William's death were of a gold standard. We were given time and space to create real and lasting memories and gently guided through the process by people who I will remember for all my life. Following William's death, I obviously went through a period of intense grief. Part of those feelings encompassed the fact I was a mum – but I was not seen as a mum because I did not have my baby. I don't intend to cause any offence by skirting over William's death ... it was the most heartbreaking time of my life but those details are another part of our story.

I found my way to cope and could understand why I felt so low, it made sense to me, my baby was dead I was allowed to be sad. My husband and I were grieving together, we picked each other up, held each other and gave each other the strength to carry on. He was ready to try for another baby before me but he waited patiently until I got there. We knew we could never replace William but we desperately wanted to be parents again.

◆ ◆ ◆

Joel

I was lucky to become pregnant again but this time I was extremely anxious during the whole pregnancy. I had a bleed at 8 weeks which I never really recovered from in terms of my anxiety. At no stage was I able to believe that the end result would be bringing a live baby home. I found it impossible to relax or have any hopes and dreams for the future. During this pregnancy, my Father in law died and he was buried beside my son, William. This formal visit to William's graveside brought about a huge resurgence of grief for me.

My second son, Joel, was born by elective section at 38 weeks. He had reflux and lost weight quickly.

I was in the hospital for over a week with him and it was during this time my anxiety turned to withdrawal and depression. It happened very quickly. My husband was shocked by the speed of my downturn but he thought that once I got home with the baby all would be well. I did not manage to sleep very much.

It took me by surprise how much Joel looked like his brother and in the wee small hours, with lack of sleep making me feel almost as if I was hallucinating, sometimes I was not sure if this baby was real, or if it was all a dream.

When we went home I continued to have difficulties breastfeeding Joel because of his reflux but I could not give up because I could not fail as a mother again by not breastfeeding successfully. I'd already failed so much as a mother, this time I HAD to do things properly. My anxiety grew and I could not accept or believe Joel was here to stay. At any point, I thought some-one would arrive to take him away. I continued to feel I was an imposter pretending to be a mum, I could not fit in with all those other "real" mums out there doing it properly. My local area began to feel hostile and unwelcoming, I did not feel safe. I began to become agoraphobic and on occasions, I had panic at-tacks. This led to me becoming socially isolated and even more lonely.

This is when I started packing and unpacking bags. At this stage, it was not too intrusive, but it sowed the seeds for something that was to become overpowering.

Eventually, I sought help from a local postnatal illness charity. I told them I was isolated, I was too ashamed and embarrassed of myself I could not admit the truth. In reality, I was suffering from depression, disrupted sleep, appetite disturbance, exhaus-tion, tension headaches, skin problems, loss of libido, anxiety, panic attacks and hair loss.

This little charity in Bristol named Mothers For Mothers was to become my refuge. It became my place of safety within my own community, in a world in which I felt I could not function. It be-came my lifeline and I credit them with saving my life and get-ting me through the suicidal thoughts that plagued me.

Through this peer support, I made friends for life. The activities and trips gave me a huge sense of relief that I was doing some-thing normal and fun with Joel and this was far easier to do with a group of women who understood how I felt.

51

◆ ◆ ◆

Trinity

When Joel was 6 months old we decided to try for another baby. I was still ill and I was terrified of being pregnant again but if we did not do it quickly I did not think I would ever have the courage. We tried unsuccessfully for 1 year. The heartache of the two-week wait followed by a negative test and the start of my cycle added to my depression. Blood tests showed I was peri-menopausal and we were referred to a fertility clinic. As we were going through the various tests I decided to stop breast-feeding Joel when he was 20 months. I fell pregnant that month — who knew?

Again I was extremely anxious during this pregnancy but this time I was also depressed and I had a toddler to care for who I felt I was letting down by not being a good enough mum. He deserved so much better than me.

When I was 6 months pregnant my own dad died. Due to my anxiety and depression, I did not have emotional space to grieve for him properly and so this was another layer of guilt to carry around. The intrusive thoughts that whenever I was pregnant someone died became very troubling.

But this time I did have more hope – I had expectations: If I was lucky enough to have another baby that lived, the postnatal illness could never be as bad because this time I would know what to expect. I would know the signs and I already had help and support in place. Little did I know...

The day after what would have been my dad's birthday, Trinity was born by elective c section at 39 weeks. The birth was traumatic. My epidural did not work properly. I was in extreme pain and I felt very alone in the theatre. The pain was so bad I did not want to hold her.

Following her birth, it was discovered that Trinity had a small hole in her heart and she underwent tests in NICU. This hit me like a brick wall. I could not look at her. If I looked at her I would love her, if I loved her she would die. I did not see a healthy baby who needed some additional support, I saw my time in NICU with William.

We did not bond and I had terrible trouble feeding her. I would not give up breastfeeding because I could not fail! I'd failed too many times at being a good mum before.

When I eventually took Trinity home, she would feed all day long. When she slept I would fall asleep while expressing another feed. She found it very difficult to latch on and I also had a toddler with IBS who I was toilet training. Every time she would be feeding comfortably he would need me for potty duty. I was a prisoner in the house. I resented my new baby because she stopped me spending time with my much longed for and dearly loved son.

I have hardly any memories of the first year of Trinity's life, every day was a struggle and there was no joy. I lost interest and enjoyment in everything. I was tearful, anxious, irritable, angry. I felt helpless, hopeless, lacking in energy and often confused. I began to have difficulties with my memory and poor concentration. I was unable to make decisions and my self-esteem was non-existent.

I was troubled with obsessive thoughts and had increasing difficulty communicating and engaging with other mums. My relationship with my husband, my family, and my friends deteriorated and I thought everyone was "against" me. The isolation and loneliness became overwhelming, like a heavy weight engulfing me, I was drowning in it, holding on by my fingertips and often I just wanted to let go and float away in the hope I could be with William again.

I thought I was a bad mum but I was obsessed with being a good mum. I was overwhelmed with guilt about how bad I really was and I was too ashamed to be honest about it. I believed that my family would be better off without me and that I was the problem. At my lowest point, I would constantly pack and unpack bags. This was intrusive to the point it began to affect my ability to parent. On one occasion I stopped the car on the motorway to unpack and repack my bag. I had no control over the urge to do this and the danger I was putting my children and others in did not hit me until after the event. This was the beginning of suicidal thoughts and plans. I thought the world would be a better place without me and that my children would be safer.

The reality of my PNI

People say treasure every moment when your children are small. The reality of my PNI is that I can't remember more than a handful of moments of my daughters first year. I remember terrible cramp in my leg after her delivery. I remember sitting in the family room outside of NICU while she was scanned. Everything else is less than a haze.

I have no idea what we did on her first Christmas Day, who we saw, what Santa brought for her, did I even shop for her presents? I don't recognise the woman with her in photographs. The woman who looked after my darling girl for a whole year. Did she love her like I do? There must have been moments of joy but she won't share them with me and I have missed so much.

This is the reality of my postnatal illness.

I have no recollection of her baptism. Was I really there? Did I choose her dress? Did I choose the roses? Did I speak to anyone? Were my friends there? Did we have fun? Did we laugh and joke? I can't remember her first word, I can't remember her first tooth, I can't remember her first steps, I can't remember what she liked to eat or what she threw on the floor in disgust!

So many memories lost ...

As Trinity grew she developed some other health problems and our relationship continued to be difficult due to our lack of bonding. I had not experienced any problems playing with Joel, in fact I had loved this time with him but I had no idea how to play or engage with Trinity.

I was obsessed with doing everything right. I would not dream of leaving the house without everything they might need for every eventuality, however, I would never have a drink or snack for myself. I did slowly begin to learn to appreciate being a mum and to enjoy time with my children. With the benefit of hindsight, I can see that I was meeting my children's needs but meeting none of my own.

Feeling low and depressed had made sense when William died, but the overwhelming feelings of anxiety and depression when I had two live babies to care for made no sense at all. During my illness it had been my choice not to take the route of medication because I was always searching for clarity, I had a need to understand what was happening to me. I also felt that I deserved to feel as bad as I did and I didn't deserve any help. It was my own fault I was a bad mother. Maybe if I had good information about medication my journey may not have been so tough and I may have recovered more swiftly. I have great respect for all women who sail these PNI seas, whatever their treatment choices, there are no easy options.

New beginnings

I had my first lucid thought on holiday a week after Trinity's first birthday, coincidental she had just given up breastfeeding by her own choice.

The children were playing in the breaking waves on the edge of the sea and I could hear them squealing with delight in the way only young children do. It was a magical sound and it was like my sense of hearing had woken up after being dulled for so long. I could not remember hearing them both laugh before. I looked at them and thought about how lucky I was, how beautiful they both were and my heart felt as if it were literally overflowing with love for them. It was the very first time I had that rush of unconditional love for Trinity. That feeling of love stopped the intrusive thoughts that had been on my mind throughout my motherhood.

From that moment onwards I promised myself I would recover. I have lovely happy memories of Trinity's second year and by her second birthday, I felt well enough to return to work after five years of illness.

During my recovery, I still had one piece of the jigsaw missing. I couldn't make sense of what had happened and my emotional responses. I stumbled upon the most beautiful, intricate, clever piece of art and everything suddenly made sense. electrical tape on the glass by Benjamin Murphy, on a building in Shoreditch.

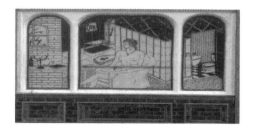

It spoke to me on another level that made me realise I had not just been carrying around my grief for William in the tiny coffin by my side but I had also been carrying around all of my dead dreams about the amazing Mother I had thought I would be. From my expected home birth to effortlessly feeding in a sling whilst doing lots of other wonderful things with my perfect babies and all the charming friends we would make.

I had expected to slip into the perfect mother role with ease and to enjoy every second. I had wanted my husband to be proud of me and to be undisturbed by the practicalities of night feeds and nappies. I had believed that my children would be perfectly well behaved and if they were not one glance from me and they would become little darlings again.

All these dead hopes, dreams and expectations together with my grief for William, my father –in –law and my dad, my grief for the person I used to be who I had completely lost in the process, were all packed in this tiny coffin that never left my side. This impacted on me every day.

I needed to say goodbye to it and to move on to the next stage of my life with my two fabulous children at my side and the memory of their brother cherished in my heart.

At last I had my clarity, my recovery was complete. Art can allow us to make sense of such intense emotions that our conscious mind attempts to protect us from. The good news is it is possible to make a full recovery from a perinatal mental illness. Like many people sometimes I have moments of anxiety and sadness. Sometimes a moment of grief about what should have been with William takes me by surprise. When I look at this picture everything makes sense again. I'm very grateful to Benjamin Murphy for the part his work played in my recovery and his gift to me of this wonderful piece of art which continues to protect my mental wellbeing. I'm in awe of such a talent that can have such a profound capacity to allow people to heal.

And finally, I am not alone. I met other amazing women who were also suffering from perinatal illness. These women continue to inspire me in the work I do. We are in union, and we not only look out for each other but we look out for the next generation of women who may need our support, and we provide that support in union together. Our children's lives have been enriched by our experiences and they have become emotionally mature.

My story finishes where it began with a gift. My inspiration and my motivation, a tiny life to honour surrounded by a mother's love.

CHEST

Hand on my chest
as you rest
close to my heart
I am held together
by stitches
in time with you

Holly Ruskin

RACHELLE

Just the baby blues?

I was never diagnosed with mental health issues before be-coming a mum but I have been seeing therapists on and off since about Middle School. I would go when I had longer periods of time being anxious or feeling really deep feelings. I would work things out with the therapist, learn tools on how to handle what I was going through and move on.

I had a hereditary predisposition for depression so I liked to make sure to go to the therapist and do maintenance on my brain when I needed it. None of those times did I ever feel as ter-rible as I did when I had postnatal depression though.

I actually even went to therapy before giving birth, concerned that PND might happen to me. When the therapist did the screening before giving birth I passed, so my worry floated away. The therapist even came to visit me after giving birth, but I didn't go back to her office until 6 months later.

Before I gave birth I was told that I would feel this overwhelming love. Yes, I loved my baby and I was excited to have him with me finally but that "all consuming love, bursts out of your chest, love," I was told about was not what I was feeling.
I felt just "ok".

Once we were home I cried. A lot.
I would get so angry when things didn't go exactly as I expected. And if something came up last minute, it meant cancelling everything else I had to do that day. I would take any excuse if it meant staying home in my PJs.

My OCD had me thinking if I didn't rock my baby precisely ten times before putting them down or if I didn't sleep facing the nursery, something terrible would happen. Not your "average" terrible, I mean out of the bloodiest horror movie terrible.

Anxiety would keep me up at night checking to make sure the baby was ok, even when I had a 24-hr nurse six days a week. The fear that something bad was going to happen wasn't a first-time mother anxious feeling; it was anxiety that would send me into full-blown panic attacks. It was so bad my chest would tighten, and I would be gasping for breath, trying to ignore it.

How could I be that anxious and be emotionally numb at the same time? I have no idea. I felt like I was failing at motherhood and I couldn't tell anyone about it because they would think terrible things of me, or even take my child from me.

Even though I had a great support group that was probably almost as afraid as I was, I felt incredibly alone.

Eventually, I was a robot going through all the motions but never truly absorbing any of the moments.

Six months after I had my son I was formally diagnosed with postnatal depression and postnatal anxiety which was also causing me to have obsessive compulsive behaviors and depersonalisation.

My PND presented itself in the form of extreme sadness, followed by emotional numbness with a hefty serving of OCD and Anxiety.

The first time I didn't ask for help for the first 6 months. The first few months I thought, it's just the baby blues, it will go away. It didn't go away. It kept getting worse.

Eventually, I got tired of crying, and I started to swallow the lump built up in my throat to avoid crying. The problem was that after swallowing my feelings for so long, my emotions just shut off.

I waited. I waited for the eight weeks I was able to breastfeed and waited for the four months I was supposed to if it was baby blues. I waited.

I remember the day it changed. I remember running to my husband and saying, "There is a boulder weighing down my emotions...I can't be as happy or even as sad as I want to be."

I loved my baby; I just wasn't able to push the rock off that love to express it outwardly. I spent almost six months locked away in my brain before I agreed to get help and take medication.

What helped me first and foremost I would say is having a support system. When I said I wasn't ok and I needed help they helped me get help. Therapy and the medications I was given were vital in my recovery. The medications helped support me while I worked with the therapist in finding other ways to support my mental health when I would have to wean-off the medication. I never needed medication before because it was just me, and therapy alone helped. This time I needed the medication to be able to function for my family, and that was ok.

When I was thinking a little clearer, I found other things that would support my emotional state once I went off the medication. I got into yoga, started taking vitamin D, and changed my diet, among other things.

Therapy taught me that I had to nourish myself before I could nourish anyone else.

I feel guilty, angry, and sad that this illness took that time away from me. That it took that time to enjoy my children when they were little (I was diagnosed with PND with both my kids). It actually blocked out memories. There are times I go back to look at pictures and realise I don't remember that moment.

I believe I still deal with the effects of PND to this day. Sometimes I find myself sitting at the edge of that black hole dangling my feet and looking at shiny objects at the bottom, wondering how far I can scoot down before I am not able to get back out. I know better now though than to go down there if I can help it.

For me I feel like I recovered from that, but I also feel like I will forever be worried. I did have another time after I had my kids when I felt that deep depression again.

I caught it in enough time though to be able to work it out with a therapist and realise what I was going through was the most extreme form of exhaustion and if I hadn't gotten the help when I did I was leading myself right back to that spot I was in with PND, and all that came with it.

So I feel like after PND I try to keep a pulse on how my brain is doing. It's like it left this mark that my brain feels it can go back to more easily than before, so I try to keep it away from that mark. I don't know if that is actually true or if the truth is that mark is something everyone has but a lot of people haven't seen inside themselves. Because I have been there and do not want to go back there again I am even more careful than before of how I am feeling and when I need help.

I have also grown so much from it. Grown as a mother, as a woman, as a person. Sometimes I am rocking at life and sometimes I am not, but I know now both are ok.

I am more in-tune with my mental health, more than ever before. I try to fill my cup full whenever, and however, I can. Not just because being happy and confident is awesome, but because I know the alternative is frightening.

I am more aware of when I am heading towards burning out, and make myself stop and find time to rest, because I know that is

one of the biggest things that affects my mental health.
I try speak up more, I am more compassionate with myself, and
I know that asking for help doesn't make me weak.

ELASTIC

Even those nights
when I've seen every hour
my heart swells and expands
elastic stretching
around the shape of you

Holly Ruskin

MOTHER

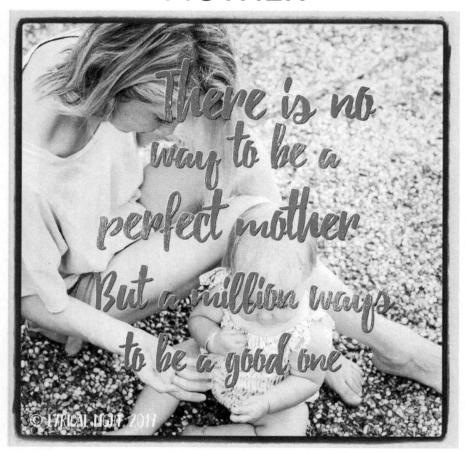

There is no way to be a perfect mother But a million ways to be a good one

© LYRICAL LIGHT 2017

CLAIRE

Running For Your Mind

Mine is a different story. I've been fortunate – a happy family, supportive husband, paid maternity leave and a career behind me, I had a lot going for me when became a mum 11 years ago. I didn't suffer with my mental well-being like many women do. But I was vulnerable like a lot of new mums.

My parents were on the other side of the world (literally!), my son was often ill and my return to work post maternity leave was full of challenges. I had to be proactive about my physical and mental health to stop me spiralling into a world of exhaustion and a mix of mental fog and overload.

I did have a bit of a head start though. I was doing my Masters in Sport and Exercise Physio at the time, and doing a dissertation on returning to activity and exercise post baby. It was this that opened my eyes to the world of postnatal depression. I was shocked to see how prevalent it was, how well documented it was in academic papers and how little was done about it in the real world. It's a widely studied fact that being physically active with others can help new mums prevent or manage postnatal depression. It surprised me that even with the knowledge that many women suffer from fluctuating moods and low moments post baby, there wasn't much more than the odd leaflet or website to help them! I think it's different for everyone, but for me, in the first few years of my children's lives, keeping up some gentle, graduated exercise was the obvious thing to do to keep me sane!

I went out walking most days with my son in the pram, and as he grew older, I did more running, set myself challenges such as 10k races. The positive sense of achievement helped me so much. Later, I joined a brilliant group called This Mum Runs. I'd always done running, swimming and other sports, and wanted to keep something of myself pre-kids. I also wanted to socialise with other mums and to get some headspace without it being all about children and whose child was showing signs of being the next child genius, junior Olympian or worse, being able to sleep through the night! I know that the baby groups in large halls work for some people, but they didn't work for me, and I'm so grateful to this group for giving me the chance to meet some amazing, inspiring and lovely women on our own terms.

Volunteering to lead group runs for This Mum Runs and later, advising them from a Physio perspective on their app, has helped me feel like I'm contributing and have something to offer other mums who might be struggling. Being an active volunteer with a mum's running community helps me connect with others and learn new skills. Giving to others and being active outside is a welcome distraction too.

I don't think it matters what it is, but it's great to have an interest outside work and home to help 'pick you up.'

MOTHERHOOD
HAIKUS

Not my only love
this mother heart is open
and you were the key

Pulled on by a string
held taut between our two hearts
tin cans to talk through

Rounded belly cut
you pulled from my open wound
a birth for us both

Cold tea and no sleep
it's hard reproducing us
even more wrinkles

Tick tock bedtime clock

RACHEL MASON

time is syrupy and slow
you sleep I creep out

I thought I would teach
but instead I learn from you
my small professor

Holly Ruskin

ROSEY

Lifting The Fog

I experienced antenatal and postnatal depression three times. That is my story in a nutshell, but for the purpose of this book I want to share my most profound experience of antenatal depression. This was with my third baby and I'm extremely lucky to still be here to share it.

At the end of 2011, I fell pregnant with my third baby, completely unplanned. It was just days before Christmas when I found out and I had two toddlers to contend with, the last thing on my mind was another pregnancy. Safe to say I was absolutely terrified when I found out. There was no joy, no excitement, simply dread at the thought of having to go through another experience of antenatal or postnatal depression.

My marriage was on its last legs, this was not the best time to be bringing another little person into our family. I sat up one night searching the internet about how to get an abortion, I couldn't imagine how I would survive another pregnancy. After a lot of soul searching, and a whole load of blind faith, I decided to continue the pregnancy. Surely it couldn't be a bad this time around? I was so wrong.

I remember telling my mum I was pregnant and her reaction was
"Oh no!", because she knew just how hard it had been for me the previous times. I kept this pregnancy quiet for a lot longer than the usual first twelve weeks, because I feared I'd end up with similar reactions from others.

So off I plodded to my booking-in appointment, duly noting down that yes, I did have a previous history of mental illness; then nothing. No additional follow ups, no referral to a mental health team. Nothing. It simply wasn't mentioned again. I was living the reality of the perinatal mental health care postcode lottery.

I hated being pregnant, I was physically, emotionally, mentally and spiritually exhausted. I would cry most days, I felt completely and utterly hopeless. There was no glowing or enjoying my growing bump. I resented everything my bump stood for. I had just started feeling mentally better after experiencing post-natal depression for the second time, so this bump was just a reminder that I could easily disappear down the dark rabbit hole of perinatal mental illness. I wasn't coping at all, I was angry at everyone, including my two young children. My life was hanging by a thread.

I didn't want to live, I had many thoughts of suicide during the pregnancy. I'm not sure what kept me going in those dark days, other than a small glimmer of hope that I had been through this before; and survived.

At 28 weeks pregnant I attended a routine antenatal appointment with a midwife. Her name was Dawn and without her, I wouldn't be sharing this story. We went through all the medical things, while chatting about how things were. I can't remember the conversation, but she could see beyond my mask, she could see I wasn't coping as well as I was trying to put across. Laughing off the exhaustion and depression, she saw right through it. She suggested I make an appointment to see my GP,
"Yes, I'll do that soon" I replied.
She knew full well I would walk out of the building and never speak to my GP. It just so happened that this appointment was in my GP surgery and she made sure I saw them before I left. This small act saved my life. I was given anti-depressants, and that lifted the fog enough for me to see that things would be ok in the end.

My baby arrived at 39 weeks. He was perfect and my experience of antenatal depression thankfully didn't affect our bond. I wore him in a sling from day one and this helped keep this experience of postnatal depression at bay, at least a little. He became my little sidekick and I am eternally grateful that Dawn the midwife saved our lives.

Through my experiences I was able to set up PND and Me, which means I can help others going through perinatal mental illness to find help, strength and to empower them to find ways to feel better. I believe everyone has within them the strength they need to overcome their experience and to live a meaningful life.

'Where there's hope, there's life. It fills us with fresh cour-

age and makes us strong again' – Anne Frank.

LUNGS

Together in the rise and fall
of your chest as you sleep
a soft echo of your time
folded under my lungs
as they breathed life into us

Holly Ruskin

IMPRINT

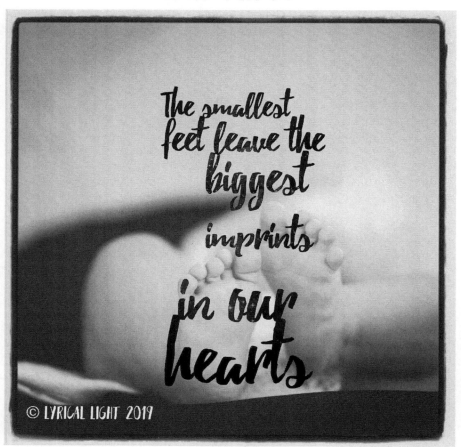

The smallest feet leave the biggest imprints in our hearts

© LYRICAL LIGHT 2019

MARK

Finding Support

H I was diagnosed with ADHD at 40 which interlinks with anxiety and low self-esteem. I self-managed it all my life without knowing it until I had a breakdown a few years after my son, Ethan was born. Having a diagnosis made my life easier and released how to manage the invisible enemy better.

Sleep is very important to me and as we know there isn't much in those early weeks. But after being a dad it just went into over-drive with so much happening in a short space of time.
I don't blame teachers but when someone tells you that you will never do anything with your life and that I wouldn't get a job it has an impact – My impact was to prove that person wrong. I have worked all my life and done everything I wanted to do from travelling the world to being a British Champion.
Self-doubt does come into my mind even today, but I know its just a thought.

I was never officially diagnosed with postnatal depression, but yes, I was suicidal four months after my boy was born. My per-sonality totally changed after his birth. I was using alcohol, while feeling anger and avoiding situations and I felt totally alone.

Witnessing my wife, Michelle go through birth trauma changed me inside as I didn't know until years later that PTSD is an anxiety disorder from either experiencing or witnessing a traumatic event. I have worked in secure units and seen so many horrible things in life but nothing worse than thinking your wife and baby are going to die in front of you.

I suffered in silence. I did not tell anyone, not even my wife Michelle. I didn't want my problems to impact on her mental health. I'd never been in a labour ward before so was naturally nervous for Michelle. I just wanted her to be OK, but not for one moment did I think we were going to be in there for more than 22 hours. With each passing hour, my anxiety was increasing. I was eager for the baby to come out and growing more worried for my wife.

Michelle was getting more tired by the hour, and I felt like a spare part. After 22 hours, there was a sense of urgency in the room and the midwives left looking worried. Shortly afterwards, doctors with no hint of expression on their faces, said the words:
"Your wife needs an emergency C-section."

I suddenly felt like I was choking and became short of breath. My heart was pounding and getting louder and louder. I thought I was going to faint. I didn't want the attention to shift to me when Michelle needed to be the priority, which made me even more uneasy. The thought of losing Michelle and our baby led me to having that first panic attack.

Thankfully, both Michelle and my son, Ethan, survived. But it became apparent a short time after the traumatic birth, that Michelle was suffering from severe postnatal depression.

Over the next few months, my personality changed as I turned to alcohol to cope, and became increasingly angry. Vivid nightmares of the birth haunted me, where Michelle and Ethan had died, and I would wake up certain that it was true. On the odd occasion where I did manage to get out and socialise with my friends, I wanted to get into fights to intentionally hurt myself and distract from the thoughts and feelings in my head. I even began to get suicidal thoughts, and couldn't seem to control them. Six months after the birth, I broke my hand punching a sofa.

Eventually I realised that as much as I wanted to be strong to look after my wife and son, the truth was that I wasn't well either. Having been brought up in a working-class community, where my father and his father before him were coal miners, all I had in my head was that I needed to "man up". I didn't feel like I could talk to anyone about it. I kept it hidden from Michelle because I didn't want to impact her mental health.
So I didn't seek help which looking back was the wrong thing to do as I always tell people "The quicker the help, the quicker the recovery"

One day something changed. I met a gentleman in the gym who went through a similar experience. I opened up and told him everything. He understood and I felt amazing for having told him. It was then I formed Fathers Reaching Out, a support group for dads looking after their partners with postnatal depression.

What is alarming was that the wife would tell me
"I'm ok but my partner is struggling after having the baby and
his struggle is impacting on my own mental health"

What I've learned from this experience is that the most important thing is that I'm a good enough father. I do make mistakes
even today but we talk and we understand it together as father
and son. Being a father is the best thing in the world and I'm
proud that my son is doing well in his life, in school and as a kind
person who wants to help people like myself and his mother.

I feel that knowing other fathers have struggled has helped me
so much. Back in 2004 when Ethan was born I thought I was the
only one who felt this way which made me feel guilty as we're
constantly told tha this should be the happiest time in our lives.

The most important thing I have learned working with parents
is that they MUST talk and ask each other if they're struggling,
looking out for any personality changes during the antenatal
and postnatal period, as it can look different in fathers.

It was the worst time of my life but it made us stronger as a
couple. After 23 years of marriage now we both work in mental health, changing our careers and not focusing on material
things to provide happiness. I have a job I just love and wake up
each day ready to go again.

Michelle's depression came back after looking after me but we
know how to seek help and know it's important to talk to each
other if you're not having a good day rather surpressing those
feeling. We know that keeping these feelings inside is more

common in men and why the biggest killer in men under 45 in the UK is suicide.

I know that my son is more likely to open up than other children as we have educated him to talk about his mental health.

Having ADHD is a disorder, so I have it for life – but I have learned mindfulness and positive coping skills which help me every day of my life. I know I need structure in my life and with wonderful friends and family I'm so lucky. I have processed everything with therapy and have purpose in my life helping health professionals to understand that perinatal mental health isn't a gender thing it can happen to ANY parent.

I have not been in that dark place for over 10 years and now know if I am doing too much. It's really important to know your triggers.

I can absolutely say that it has changed me for the better and I have more empathy for people who are struggling with their mental health.

In 2012, I was awarded Inspirational Father Of The Year and Local Hero at the Pride Of Britain Awards. On World Mental Health Day in 2016 I was invited to meet The Royal Family and in 2019 I was awarded the Point Of light Award by the Prime Minister.

I'm also an Ambassador for the Mothers For Mother's Charity.
I always wanted something positive to come out of something so bad. I am now a published author of two books, written journals with Dr Jane Hanley, campaigned around the world, spoken on television and radio globally and found my passion in life to help parents and change policy by publishing a new report.

What we want is advocacy, screening and better support for new fathers as I feel it's a missing piece of the jigsaw. When ALL parents are supported in their mental health it has far better outcomes for the whole family and the development of the child. We also know it can impact on the mothers mental health if the father is not supported and there is more drinking, avoidance of situations and anger, so we know that providing support for dads will save many relationships too.

Mental health early prevention should start during pregnancy for parents as it's so important in those first 1001 Critical Days.

LOVE

Love
light and feathered
she is there
as I watch you sleep
settled in my heart
listening to your tiny sighs
she is with me
in the darkest nights
love never leaves me now
when I can't see another day
it is love's hand at my back
keeping me as I keep you
in all things now I look to her
and know the storms
they are weathered
she is there
love

Holly Ruskin

ELISE

Breathing Space

"What's your birth plan?"
I remember being asked this question all the time during my pregnancy. I was given leaflets about antenatal testing, scans, eating healthily during pregnancy, midwife appointments, prenatal vitamins, how to write a birth plan, what to expect during the stages of labour. My friends also recommended hypnobirthing and we went on the course, all to help us prepare for the birth of our child.

But not one person said anything to me about what happens after...

I never thought I would suffer with my mental health after having a baby. I'll admit I was incredibly naive and often assumed that people either weren't trying hard enough or weren't as caring if they struggled after having a child. TV and social media only make this worse, showing mothers taking to it naturally, smiling in all their perfect family photos, sharing posts such as "he/she is my world" or "never been so happy and in love". You never realise that behind those posts is a woman who hasn't slept properly for weeks or even months, doesn't have time to shower, is at the beck and call of another human 24 hours a day, doesn't ever get time alone to even drink a cup of tea, and is despairing. Since going through my own experiences I vowed to be as honest as possible with people, because it was other people's honesty that got me through when things weren't going great.

I'd suffered with intermittent anxiety in the past, having had two or three incredibly dark and scary patches in my life. However the couple of years leading up to having my daughter I was managing the anxiety well and had very few episodes, so even though I knew it was possible, I thought I would be ok. I'd suffered two miscarriages before my daughter was born, and wanting to have a child absolutely consumed me, so I believed I would appreciate and enjoy every second when it did arrive.

My daughter's birth was fairly traumatic. We'd done hypnobirthing and I was fully planning for a calm, intervention-free birth. We ended with the complete opposite. Complications late in the pregnancy meant I was strongly advised to have an induction, which lasted three days and led to an emergency caesarean when my daughter got into distress. Saying I was exhausted was an understatement, I was vomiting from sheer weakness and crying because I thought I was going to drop my baby on the floor.

What I needed, and what my head needed, was rest.

Staying in hospital was hard on the ward. My daughter had an episode where she choked on the fluid in her lungs, and after that was diagnosed with jaundice. Once being discharged we had to go back into hospital every 12 hours to check her jaundice levels and have a heel prick test. I remember her screaming in pain and feeling her pain shoot through me. I can still feel that feeling now when I think back to it.

I left the hospital, bone-tired, worrying about my daughter's jaundice. I remember getting in the car and as soon as my husband pulled away I suddenly went cold and panicked thinking "they can't let me take her home, I have no idea what to do, I can't keep her alive!" - this was where the anxiety started. I walked through the door and just cried. This wasn't the rush of love I'd been promised. I was too exhausted to feel anything other than shock.

I think the exhaustion mixed with the trauma of the birth was the main factors to developing postnatal anxiety. Because of the jaundice my daughter was very sleepy and so rarely completed a feed, and was asleep on me all of the time. I couldn't ever just put her down like all the books suggested, so those early weeks consisted of me staying up all night with her on me, terrified to close my eyes. My husband wanted to help as much as possible but I wanted to breastfeed so meant she was on me all the time. And although I trust him, I was so anxious he would also fall asleep with her on him, and I just couldn't hand her over at night time. I started to develop severe anxiety and dread about the nights.

A few days after we arrived home we went to a friend's daughter's first birthday party. I was so tired, but I wanted to prove to myself that we could get out of the house, and felt guilty at the prospect of cancelling. After everyone had left I was sitting on the sofa with my friend and she turned to me and said
"you're doing so much better than I was at this stage. It was

awful for me".

She then opened up to me about her experiences with mental health and I was just amazed. It was the first time someone had told me they struggled, and it suddenly lifted a weight off my shoulders to know that I wasn't alone.

My anxiety sky rocketed over those first few weeks. I couldn't eat, any food I did have just tasted like charcoal and I lost about a stone in three weeks. As a result my milk supply suffered, which caused more mental health problems. I was exhausted beyond belief but was so terrified of falling asleep with my daughter on me as I'd been told so many times that she would slip onto the cushions and suffocate. It just seemed to snowball and I found I just wanted to escape. I desperately wanted some-one to come and take her for a bit, so I could just have some breathing space. I couldn't even have a bath as every time she squeaked I felt a rush of adrenaline and raced out to get to her. I felt that so much was expected of me as the mother, that I was supposed to just take to this naturally and find it all a breeze. I just didn't and I spent all of the time thinking there was some-thing wrong with me. I thought I wasn't fit to be a mother and that I mustn't love my daughter because I felt this way.

I remember feeling so jealous of my husband. After his two week paternity leave he went back to work. Although I always appre-ciated that he had work to do, and he wasn't there for fun, I was still so jealous that he could go and spend 8 hours sitting in peace, drinking tea whenever he wanted to, he could laugh and chat with his colleagues. All the while I was stuck at home struggling just to leave the house. Before I got pregnant I had bought tickets for us to see a comedian in Bristol. Our daughter was born three weeks before the show so I couldn't go and my husband went with his brother. I remember sobbing and sob-bing that evening, thinking I would never be able to enjoy that part of my life again.

Looking back all of this makes me terribly sad. If only I'd known back then just how normal it was, I don't think I'd have struggled nearly as much. If only I'd known just how much I did love my daughter, and would grow into my role, perhaps I would've been kinder to myself. I really appreciated my friend who'd spoken out to me in those early days, and after I started reaching out to people and talking about how I was feeling more and more people came back saying just how much they'd struggled. I now make it my mission to be honest with people, to encourage them to talk about how they're feeling and to support them.

The turning point was when we saw a breastfeeding consultant, she said that if the mother can get four hours of uninterrupted sleep, then she can survive the rest of the day. I had been getting much less than that up until then. That evening at 5pm my husband insisted I go upstairs, put ear plugs in, and not to come downstairs until he woke me. At midnight he woke me up. I'd slept for seven hours solidly, I just cried with relief when I realised how long I'd slept. Over the next weeks this became our routine, by that point we were combination feeding with a bit of formula and it helped me to gain the energy and strength I needed to recover.

We were very fortunate that our daughter started sleeping well from quite early on, and even though breastfeeding was a huge struggle for us I persevered and at about 11 weeks it suddenly clicked and became easier. It was the longest eleven weeks but everything started to calm down, even though I was struggling and still wanted to be by myself from time to time. I've started to realise this is normal - we all need breathing space, regardless of what stage of life we are in.

I was never officially diagnosed with a postnatal mental health condition, but I did talk openly with my health visitor, and they made additional regular visits to check in. I found the local community midwives and health visitors were very supportive at the time.

I have recovered from the anxiety, but I do still have moments where I don't enjoy motherhood, I think we all do, and that's normal. It's incredibly hard and it's permanent. You don't just hand the baby back at the end of the day. For me, the main way I cope is by having regular things to look forward to. We are lucky to have a very supportive family network around so are able to have days out, and the occasional night away.

When your baby is born, it is so intense and sudden. There is no gentle introduction into parenting, it hits you at the hardest point. You often feel you have lost part of yourself and you grieve the old life that you used to have. The freedom and the space to be by yourself when you want. However what I didn't realise back then is that as the weeks and months go by, the old you starts to return. You find your feet, you may decide to go back to work, you will be able to leave your child with others and go out and enjoy yourself, and when you do you will enjoy it even more.

Nothing will ever change your life in the same way as having a baby. Nothing can prepare you for it and if you don't enjoy the changes immediately, it doesn't mean you don't love your child. You will grow, you will adapt, and you will love your child more than you could ever know. You just need to give it time.

FLOWERS

Your love
draws us close
no sliver of space
whisper or sigh between
we are two pressed flowers

Holly Ruskin

BORN

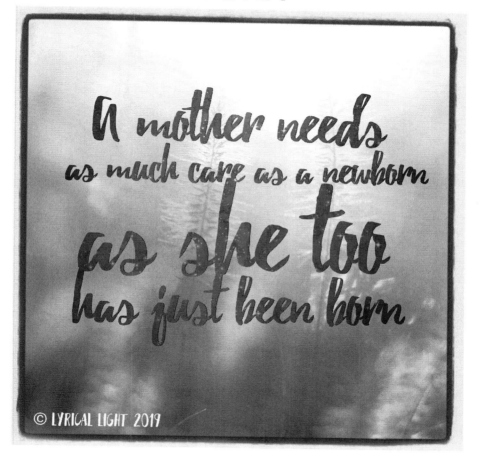

A mother needs
as much care as a newborn
as she too
has just been born

© LYRICAL LIGHT 2019

JESMINDER

Anxiety Blinkers

I have always been an anxious person, with my anxiety fluctuating over time. A few years ago several life events happened at once and I found myself feeling highly anxious with frequent panic attacks. After a few weeks of this I also started to feel low in mood, because I was so fed up of anxiety and avoidance behaviours controlling how I lived my life. I had counselling but have never had any kind of diagnosis.

During pregnancy and after birth I felt such love for my son that, although I felt huge relief he had been born safely, I felt great anxiety that something was going to go wrong. There was nothing even remotely as important as making sure everything went "well" for him. He had a couple of choking episodes on mucus in his first few days, once when he was lying down. From that point we decided he just couldn't be horizontal- not very practical for a baby! So we held him day and night for the first few weeks. This can't have helped my mental health!

In the weeks and months that followed I feel I bonded with him to such an extent that I couldn't pay attention to anything else.

Showering away from him would cause me anxiety. My own health also caused me worry because passing blood clots and feeling debilitated by mastitis left me too anxious/unwell to care for him. This was only ever for a matter of hours but I felt I needed to be there for him every minute of the day. I was obsessed with his temperature, monitoring his clothing and room temperature, whether he was developing a rash, how much milk he'd had, the consistency of every nappy. I didn't want anyone else to distract from that, and I felt I didn't provide him "optimum" care when friends and family came to visit. I found the majority of visits extremely stressful, and would spend most of the time on the boundaries of where anxiety turns into a panic attack.

The people around me who'd had babies at a similar time seemed much more confident as parents, and were able to go out and socialise with their babies happily, while I found it extremely stressful to be away from home with my baby.

I spoke to the health visitors about my mental health at one of the clinic appointments. She said I was scoring on the anxiety scale, but not for depression. I was given a number to self refer for phone CBT if I wanted it. Again, I have never had a diagnosis. I did find some benefit with the phone service, although I think as time went on things improved naturally. The main thing that changed for me was that once I had experienced something perceived as "negative" and handled it well, I felt more confident doing it a second time. Gradually I came to believe that I could handle more situations than I thought I could. I also feel as I got to know my baby more I could more intuitively tell whether he was ill or what was wrong, without my thought process being led by anxiety.

I certainly feel I have recovered from how I felt at that time. I now feel like a better version of myself who has occasional periods of heightened anxiety and infrequent panic attacks. While I have forgotten the finer details of the birth and it has become "rose-tinted", I haven't forgotten how awful I felt during those first months. I'm so happy to feel like I can fully enjoy motherhood and spending time with my son now. It's like I have taken the anxiety blinkers off!

EYES

The way I see it now
is through your eyes
the ones that look like mine
and that makes me want to swim
against the tides and
howl
at every moon
forge all my paths
go against each tiny grain
push
back and be like
the slickest
oil
in water
sing out of tune and
run
up that hill
stick out
like the sorest thumb
be the farthest cry and
stand out in the largest crowd
and blow against the wind
all while writing
my own story
to show you
that

RACHEL MASON

we can

Holly Ruskin

FAITH

Happy To Still Be Here

A long time before I became a mum I had been through a really traumatic and volatile relationship which led me to develop anxiety and depression. This was from emotional, physical and mental abuse and when that relationship ended the remnants of that stayed with me. A relationship like that is not something you can just recover from, you have to grow and heal and make yourself better, which is what I did.

After giving birth I was elated, joyous and overwhelmed. I think after all three of my births I had every feeling imaginable. You're up and down for weeks, thinking am I doing it right? Am I making the most of my baby being so small, as everyone tells you that's what you should do. Then I felt drained after a couple of weeks and I couldn't pick myself up, mentally I was null and void.

I felt lost, lonely and scared but I also felt happy. I was so up and down, one minute crying under the table because I wasn't doing it well enough and the next I was in baby swimming classes smashing it with my 6 week old. There's no one single feeling to describe you after birth.

The first time I went to the doctors after my first child it was labelled "baby blues" and something I'd get over. With my second child it came back so I just put it down to the same thing and carried on. Then came baby number three and I was broken, suicidal, experiencing psychosis and couldn't leave the house. It turns out that postnatal depression hadn't been diagnosed after my first child was born so just continued over three and a half years until it hit me like a steam train.

Eventually I asked for help in June 2019, four months after baby number three and only because my partner made me talk to my health visitor. I received counselling from her but in November I took an overdose in an attempt to take my own life as my psychosis had taken over without me speaking up properly. I just said what people wanted to hear to make it go away.

After the overdose I had to wait a long time. It was a case of strong tablets that made me into a zombie. In March just before lockdown I made the decision to come off my tablets (instant feeling of lightness) and seek private counselling as NHS funded waiting lists are insanely long. I have been having weekly zoom calls with my counsellor, eating healthily and exercising which is helping me greatly.

When I think back over that time I know how far I've come, but I'm aware I'm still very much in it. I look back to my worst days with fear, fear it could come back like it was.

I don't really feel I'm fully recovered yet. I'm not fully there. I still have suicidal thoughts, days where my psychosis is bad but I'm having more good days than bad so it's working.

I feel completely changed by this. I'm getting the old me back but with a twist. I'm scared, anxious and fearful but I'm also grateful, intrigued and happy to still be here.

GUILT

Motherhood means
no relief or reprieve
from doing my best
so I crave those days
when I failed
only myself
and guilt didn't linger
but we simply passed
like ships in the night

Holly Ruskin

WAITING WITH YOU

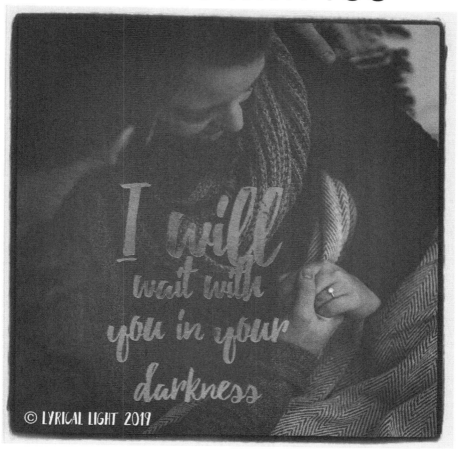

© LYRICAL LIGHT 2019

MICHAL

Like All Things, This Will Pass

I am a type-A, over-achieving introvert, and much of my life satisfaction has been dependent upon my achievements. Straight-A student, major label recording artist, Emmy winner, corporate lawyer, you get the gist.

When I got pregnant at 29, I threw myself into motherhood with the same intensity, but my pregnancy coincided with a lot of upheaval. We moved to a suburbia, far (literally and figuratively) from the manic creative energy of New York City, which my brain is a mirror for. I was unmoored. I gave birth at home and nearly died from postpartum hemorrhage. (Sidebar: it was idyllic until the end, and our midwife was extremely prepared and saved my life).

In the twilight period following my first son's birth I was severely anemic, struggling to breastfeed and waking at all hours. I remember the creeping feeling of unease as the sun began to set, knowing what lay ahead. In my moments of sleep I would dream of changing the baby, and then I would wake and do it; a constant Groundhog Day loop. When my baby was a year old, I was pregnant again. And two years later, I was pregnant with my third son. I never gave myself the space or time to process what

I had voluntarily given up.

I have never had a lot of close friends, and my husband had no personal experience with depression or anxiety. He eventually became exhausted from being my main emotional support and withdrew, pushing me into therapy and to take antidepressants, which didn't work for me.

I was a high functioning depressive, because "doing" kept me from thinking too much. I dropped to 95 pounds. I felt like I was at the bottom of a well and I couldn't see a way out.

The things that helped me return to myself were, ultimately: long walks through graveyards at night (very dramatic, I know). Writing music as a way of siphoning off the poison-over one hundred songs, that poured out of me, compulsively, 14 of which became my album "No Resolution," a brutally honest snapshot of that moment in time. Reconnecting with an old friend who was also suffering from depression and talking each other through it, hundreds of hours of conversations between the damned. My children, for whom I knew I had to recover. And time. Eventually, like everything, it passed.

The things that didn't help were the forced interventions. The pathologising of a normal and common experience. I was afraid that if people really knew what I was going through they would question my fitness to parent, to teach music, to care for myself.

My goal in writing this is to hopefully make it easier for others to seek and give constructive support. If it takes a village to raise a child, mothering cannot be a solitary act. No mother

RACHEL MASON

should be left alone at the bottom of a well.

HUE

If I lived
in my love for you
there'd be no cool tones
just the warmest of hue

Holly Ruskin

BIANCA

I Am Free

To be me, to be free.

To be me, to be free, that's all I want to be. Thinking back to way before having my boys, but to after leaving school. They were 'my best years'. I was home taught for the last 2 years of school due to depression, which then seemed to disappear as I started working. My best years were spent working 3 jobs at once, laughing, singing, going out with friends. Fast forward 5 years and I fell pregnant with our first boy, George. The anxiety crept in.

Looking back now I'd say it was because I wasn't working, getting out, talking to anyone 'on the outside world' other than my fiance Ben and family. I would struggle socially. Then having George, the intrusive thoughts became worse. There were times I couldn't even let family hold him. I had to leave the room to stop myself asking them to get off my baby. As he grew older my anxiety settled.

Falling pregnant with Roman struck it up again, even worse. Yet as soon as I had Roman it was like a light switch turning my anxiety off. A faulty light switch that turned itself back on after a couple of months. This time 10 times worse. These were the worst times, when 'my monster' unleashed itself. I called it my monster because it was like something taking over my body, mentally, physically and emotionally. Sometimes it would last hours, and afterwards I could barely remember it happening.

It took me 5 years to actually ask properly for help from someone other than Ben. In fact, in the end it was Ben that had to ring our local crisis team for me. I'd tried numerous times with the doctor and midwives. During my second pregnancy I was referred to a midwife who specialises in mental health. I'm still waiting for her to call 2 years on. I feel this needs to be worked on more with health professionals so they're able to substantially support people who are suffering with mental health.

I wish I had demanded help sooner, but the anxiety took over so much. When I was younger with depression I had tried counselling, but it didn't work for me. And I felt tablets would take over me, but I knew there was no other way. I couldn't keep living like that. I've tried 3 different anxiety tablets, it's the best thing I've ever done. I'm not ashamed to say I have anxiety and I'm on medication for it.

As my anxiety crept back after having Roman that's where Mum For The Sons started on Instagram. It gave me something to focus on and somewhere to get things off my chest. Since then I've set up a separate page for my mental health posts. My aim is to help others struggling, help others to understand mental health and contribute towards ending the stigma. I completely get that if you don't suffer with mental health it's very difficult to understand it, as it is even for those who do suffer.

My Instagram has been a massive help for me, as well as me helping others. Also music helps to ease my anxiety. In my teens I
used to listen to music nearly all day everyday. Since having the
boys the only music that would be on is cbeebies or Ben's music
until my Dad bought me an Alexa for Christmas. Now whenever
I feel myself getting worked up with emotions I put my music
straight on and it instantly relaxes my mood and tension.

I don't feel recovered, I still have bad days (everybody does) but
nowhere near as bad as they were. I'm learning how to manage it
a lot better and be the one in control. My daily mirror ritual in
the beginning was,
"I am me, I am free, I own my anxiety."
It may sound silly, you may feel stupid, but it worked for me.
Look deep into your eyes to the real you.

If you're struggling or know someone that is, it can be extremely hard to 'just talk to someone.' But I beg you to please do
rather than suffer in silence. You are definitely not alone.
From opening up about my own struggles on my Instagram
account, I've had quite a few people message me how they're
struggling just the same and we have helped each other through
the hard times. So even if you feel you can't talk to your family,
friends or doctor, drop me a message!

You're not being a burden by opening up.

IN

*My cracks
let your
love
in*

Holly Ruskin

ONE BREATH CLOSER

Words falling through me
Like sand through the glass.
I know what you'd say
That this too shall pass.

Rachel Mason
Dedicated to my mother, Jackie and mother-in-law, Maggie.

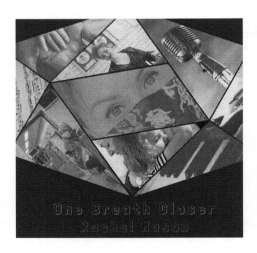

SAMARA

Learning To Have A Voice

I n 2009 I was a young 27 years old when I became a mum. I thought I knew everything I needed to know about birth. I had watched my sister being born and I read all the pregnancy and birth books.

I felt so special during my first pregnancy. The spotlight was on me and everyone was excited waiting for the new arrival. I was at that prime age of when friends were getting married and having children.

Early one morning, at 5am to be exact, I felt like I needed to pee. As I turned to get out of bed, I felt a big gush and I knew it was time. I was exactly 40 weeks pregnant. Hours passed and we had even been to the hospital to check me over. Not much was happening with labour just yet.
"Come back tomorrow morning" the midwife said "and we will assess what we will do with you."

As the night went on a few contractions came and went but nothing was regular. The next morning we ventured back to the hospital around 8am. As we sat in the waiting room for a birthing room to become available we were told I was to be induced at about 10am.

Soon after I was seen too, all the action started. I was hooked up to a drip, fetal monitor and about 20 minutes later I started to feel the contractions starting and then becoming regular. Once we were all ready for the baby to arrive, I was 'checked' to see how dilated I was and I was 3cm. I thought to myself... not bad doing that all on my own so far.

I felt like while I was induced it's all about clock watching and fetal monitoring. About three hours after being checked the first time, it was time for another routine 'check' from the midwife and doctor to see how I was progressing. As this was happening my husband said to me that I should be about 6 or 7 cms now, because that's what they told us in birthing class. One centimetre dilation per hour. So when the midwife said... Hmmm still 3cm dilated, I was devastated. I'd had enough. I didn't want to be doing this anymore.

The next few hours were a blur, contractions got more intense and I was using the gas to get me through them. I felt like I was in a different place when I was sucking on the gas. During this time I do remember the midwife fussing about with the fetal monitor realising it wasn't really working properly so we weren't getting a very good reading on the baby.

I don't know what time it was by this stage. I was in a lot of pain with contractions and was starting to demand pethidine for pain relief. Then the midwife appeared with a new fetal monitor and brought it into the room. She got it hooked up and got the measurements of the baby's heart rate then the midwife suddenly left the room to get another midwife.

I started vomiting from using the gas as it was up too high. At this stage I was yelling or crying, I can't remember which one it was now, at my husband for the pethidine. The midwife explained that we needed to wait as the baby's heart rate is dropping with every contraction. It was decided very quickly to turn off the drip that was inducing these contractions. She checked my cervix and I was still only 3cm dilated. She suggested that an emergency c-section was a really good option right now. She was waiting for the surgeon to come in and check my chart.

I remember the surgeon coming into the birthing room looking at my chart and asked me if I was happy to proceed with an emergency c-section. I said yes and this overwhelming feeling of relief came over me with the thought that I didn't have to do this anymore. As we left the room I looked at the clock and it was just before 6pm. I was being wheeled into surgery with the medical team with me, signing papers of consent along the way.

Everything happened so quickly, some parts are still really blurry. And like a click of the fingers my baby was born at 6.32pm and a healthy good size baby boy.

He was placed in a humidicrib and once the surgery was all done I was in recovery where my body went into shock. I was shaking and so cold. But I didn't have my baby with me. The midwife had taken him up to the maternity ward and my husband followed to where my mum, stepdad and little sister were all waiting and excited to meet my new baby.

This is the bit that gets me every time and I love my family to the moon and back. But I wasn't the first one to hold my baby. My family all got to kiss and cuddle him. I missed out on skin to skin contact and our first breastfeed after birth. I finally got to hold my baby boy just over two hours after he was born. To me this whole experience was traumatic. I took a long time to bond with my baby and I honestly believe that because we didn't get that skin to skin and breastfeeding time right after birth.

I've had three more sons since this experience, all c-sections. But I can tell you that each birth has been very different from the others. I found the recovery from 'elective' c-section is much easier than an emergency c-section.

One thing I did learn and that I made very clear to the hospital was that I was to have my baby with me in recovery at all times, to have skin to skin contact and have that opportunity to breastfeed. These moments were so important to me.

When I think of my traumatic birth experience I can now talk about it, knowing that I have done some work with healing. Looking at the situation and being first time parents we honestly didn't know what was happening or why. One thing I am thankful for in this whole experience is that I learned to have a voice and to use it. Any mum I come across who is willing to discuss or ask questions, I simply tell them to be aware of different outcomes that can happen in birth. Don't just have one birth plan. Have a plan in place for vaginal birth and c-section birth. One thing I wish I had especially for when I had my first son is a postnatal Doula. Someone there a few hours a day with me and the baby to help us work it all out together.

Breastfeeding is so natural but it doesn't come easy. I have to admit I never had a good enough milk supply with all my babies and all four of my sons had to be supplemented with formula, which resulted in them being formula fed. I love the motto of "fed is best". Because there is one thing I learned through new-born babies is that if they are happy and content they will sleep well, and so will you.

Birth for me hasn't changed me as a person, but becoming a mother certainly has. It does. A mother is also born when her baby is and while we are learning to look after this new human that we have created, we too have changed. This is something that isn't spoken about all too often. We need to nurture the new mother as much as the newborn baby. There is so much build up during the pregnancy to holding your baby in your arms, but what happens next? I felt this in the most recent time going through my own life journey of rediscovering who I am other than just mum.

What I have learned is that I am more than mum. We can be anything. Honestly. I feel that mothers hold onto perfectionism way too much and this causes us to hide away from the outside world. Let's be honest. Life with kids is messy. Motherhood is messy. There is no perfect way. There is only your way. Do what works for you, that's all that matters at the end of the day. You are more than you think you are.

KNOWING

Love goes to the edge
and pours itself over
not held or contained
but a rushing power
the roar we hear
before the hush
storm before the calm
the deafening noise
and then the quiet knowing
that sits in all our hearts

Holly Ruskin

RACHEL

The Darkness Behind
The Stage Lights

My first few days as a first time mum were a blur. I remember feeling intense love for my little baby girl but such overwhelming fear and unhappiness too. I didn't know if this was normal and felt too afraid to ask in case the answer was

"No. Other people don't feel like this. It's just you."

I hoped it was just the much talked about "baby blues" and that it would pass in a couple of days but as time went on I realised it was something more, something darker, something that was bigger than me and at times felt bigger than the immense love I had for my daughter.

A frantic midnight Google search with tears in my eyes confirmed my fears. It was postnatal depression. I had suffered from depression years before and had been gently warned by the midwife during my pregnancy that I was statistically more likely to have postnatal depression if I'd had depression before.

I vividly remember looking in the mirror and saying to myself "I will not let myself have postnatal depression. I'll beat the statistics"

Now I look back at that thought I feel so foolish. No amount of my usual unswerving determination could control what was happening to me. For the next few months the waves of emotion came and went without warning and I refused to talk to anyone about it in case they confirmed my worst fears that I was crazy and decided that my little girl should be taken away from me.

During this time I was asked to be an expert judge for the brand new Sky One show Sing: Ultimate A Cappella. It was going to be hosted by Cat Deeley and would feature a cappella groups from across the UK and Ireland competing to win the approval of the judges.

I loved filming the show, working with the other judges, meeting pop stars and hearing some fantastic a cappella performances but behind the dazzling stage lights, make up and tv glamour I felt like I was drowning. My job was to paint on a smile and make sure the producers didn't regret their decision choosing me for the judging panel. Confronting the darkness inside me would have to wait. And wait it did.

It's only really when the show aired three months later and friends commented on how I seemed to "have it all together", taking my career and motherhood in my stride that I felt like a huge fraud. I didn't have it all together at all and the fragile shell I had made around myself started to crack. I started secretly self harming to try and control what I could not control, but it soon became clear that this wasn't going to be enough.

Finally, 6 months after the birth I reached breaking point and reached out to my health visitor for help. She advised Talk Therapy which helped a lot. I also told my husband, immediate family and close friends how I had been feeling for the last few months. They all said they were so relieved I had spoken to them. They said they knew something was wrong but didn't know how to talk to me about it as I was so shut down.

A few months after weekly Talk Therapy I was feeling much more like myself again. My husband and I decided we'd like to have another baby and talked a lot about how I'd struggled with postnatal depression after our first baby. It was the first time I'd really shared with him how bad it had been and he was overwhelmingly loving and supportive.

I had a touch of antenatal depression with our second child and hoped that would be the extent of it, but the postnatal depression kicked in hard the day after I gave birth. However, I was determined for things to be different this time and asked for help, visiting my doctor and being prescribed antidepressants.

This decision changed everything. I still had to work to try and shake off the stigma of "mental health issues" but allowing myself to be honest about my feelings and accept support, both emotional and medical has meant I've had an easier journey with my second child.

If you're struggling with symptoms of antental or postnatal depression I urge you to speak to someone. Please don't leave it as long as I did.

STRANGER

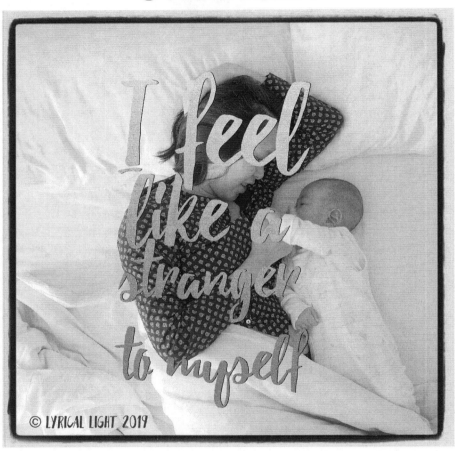

© LYRICAL LIGHT 2019

TIGHTER

Holding you tighter
always comes
when I know it's time
to let you grow

Holly Ruskin

AMY

One Tuff Muvva

I didn't feel great during my pregnancy, physically or mentally. I wasn't happy about being pregnant and however much I tried, I couldn't get excited. I felt an impending sense of doom and the feeling that my life was over.

I didn't share how I was feeling with anyone as I felt guilty and didn't think they'd understand. I tortured myself with guilt as so many people want children and can't have them yet there I was dreading becoming a mother. I kept thinking to myself that everything would be ok once she's here.

When Maddie was born, she was handed to me and I waited for the rush of love but it didn't come. I told myself that I loved her but I felt nothing. I had a sickening, claustrophobic feeling that this was my life now. It felt like a weight pressing down on my chest and I felt an overwhelming sense of regret at becoming a parent.

The first night at home was awful. Maddie screamed non-stop and I was convinced that she would die from my lack of maternal instinct. I had been awake for over 96 hours and was extremely on-edge. I was frantically googling EVERYTHING and making myself sick with worry.

The midwife came round the next morning and I couldn't control my tears. I was told that it was just 'baby blues'. I told her that I didn't want to be a Mum. She sent me back to hospital.
Back in hospital, I was told that how I was feeling was 'normal' and I needed to try and get some rest. I felt so stupid. I was so anxious. I was starting to realise that this wasn't just 'baby blues', I wanted to die. Like, actually end my own life right that second.

The midwife came to check on me and I kept asking her to end my life. I was sobbing and saying this over and over again. Doctors came in to tell me that everything was going to be ok. I didn't believe them. I had reverted back to being a child again. I felt vulnerable and unable to function as an adult let alone a parent. Every little thing was a struggle.
I felt so unbelievably low and desperate. It was the worst feeling I had ever felt and I couldn't see it getting any better.

I was tired of caring so much about what others thought of me. Tired of hating myself so much. I thought that everyone would be so much better off without me. I saw my opportunity and ran for the door with the intention of ending my life. I wanted the pain to stop once and for all. I ran for the exit but was tackled by a midwife.

I was sectioned under section 4 of the Mental Health Act for my own safety. This meant I couldn't leave the hospital for 72 hours. I was assessed by doctors and psychiatrists and it was decided that I was very unwell and was placed in a Mother and Baby Unit 3 hours away from home.

I was petrified and had to be sedated for the journey. We arived at the MBU and I was assessed at 1am. I was exhausted, distraught and drowsy from the sedative. I was sectioned again.

This time under section 2 which meant I could be detained for up to 28 days. I became very distant from Maddie and didn't want to be near her. Every little sound or movement she made triggered my anxiety. I constantly told myself that life was good and many people have it worse. Which just added to the guilt. You cannot talk yourself out of depression. Just like you cannot talk yourself out of having the flu or a broken leg.

I was exhausted though I wasn't doing much apart from existing. I had no appetite and didn't enjoy anything anymore. I felt like I was living in a dark hole with no escape. Making decisions was difficult. I didn't like thinking about the future as it seemed so grey. I didn't believe that I would ever feel better but slowly, with the help of family, friends and professionals, I learned to let go of the guilt and accept that I had an illness. I was then able to really begin my recovery.

Intrusive thoughts became less frequent and my emotions levelled out. I was trying hard to bond with Maddie and would take her out for walks by myself. One day it dawned on me that I was enjoying spending time with her instead of fearing it. I finally felt like the clouds were clearing.

I am much better now and am proud of how far I have come. I have worked hard at my recovery and kept going when all I wanted to do was disappear.

My advice is please don't suffer in silence. Accepting help was the best thing I ever did.

Remember that you are NOT alone and there are people out there that want to help you too!

I decided to launch One Tuff Muvva after I had already spearheaded 2 successful mental health
campaigns through my role as a senior graphic designer at Funky Pigeon. I felt the time had come to
create a platform that was completely separate. I wanted to create a platform that gave people
hope and made them feel good whilst acknowledging the seriousness of mental ill health. I wanted
it to be as interactive as possible and for people to feel as if they could reach out to me if needed.

After nearly losing my life to this horrible illness, I wanted to create a safe space for others going
through similar experiences. A place to share awareness and experience as well as hope and
positivity.

I create illustrations and quotes for my grid of things that have helped or resonated with me in the
past and try and accompany these with something personal/helpful in the captions. I only ever post
when I feel that I have something important or helpful to share and I really don't have a clue (or
care!) about algorithms etc! If one of my posts can help just one person then I feel that it has served
it's purpose. My stories are filled with more of my personal life ie. Funny things that my daughter
has said/done etc. I hope that by posting these kind of stories, I can give hope to women who may
be suffering that they too, can share the same bond with their child despite how they may feel right
now. I also have a website with free resources such as the Mental Health Toolkit for people to download and a shop with little

RACHEL MASON

gifts that I have designed to make it easier to send a small gift to someone who may be struggling.

FEEL LIKE YOU

When you're feeling lost
In life's deep rolling waves
Hold on to the life raft
And look to calmer days.

No, nothing lasts forever
I promise you
We'll face this storm together
And you'll come through.
You'll reach the shore again
You'll feel like "you" again.

When you're feeling rested
And close the door to fear
Feel the warmth upon you
For brighter days are here.

Rachel Mason

HEART

Blood and bone you are
the heart outside my chest
beating every minute
and in this shortest of seasons
you are all I hear

Holly Ruskin

HELEN

Never Stop Taking Care Of Yourself

I remember reading a quote once that said, 'the most natural state of motherhood is unselfishness. When you become a mother you are no longer the centre of your own universe. You relinquish that position to your children'

I think most of us would agree that our children become the centre of our world and that is a beautiful thing; to love another so deeply. But all too commonly as we enter motherhood, we forget to take care of ourselves in the way we deserve. In our eagerness to be the perfect mum - to do things right - we get consumed by the needs of our child, and our own self-care falls by the way-side.

This 'striving for perfection' began even before my daughter was born. I always believed giving birth could be a wonderful experience and was determined to birth my baby, without unnecessary medical intervention or drugs. Despite achieving this goal, when my daughter emerged I was exhausted, disorientated and then had to endure an hour of surgery and a blood transfusion; separated from my newborn I missed out on the 'golden hour' and was unable to bond.

My postnatal recovery was very slow and I felt I was falling well-short of the mother I wanted to be. I found it hard to leave my daughter's side and if I wasn't constantly entertaining her with some activity or group, I would feel guilty. I would strive to make her the most nutritious homemade food and kept a close watch on whether she was getting enough sleep and at the right time. My husband was always out at work early and rarely home before her bedtime and I had no family support locally, so it was tough trying to do most of the parenting on my own. I never felt I could ask for help or let others know how miserable and exhausted I felt, because I thought it would be an admission of failure. I loved my daughter deeply but felt so alone and like there would never be any respite from the early waking and broken nights.

I continued to breastfeed my daughter for nearly two years, but I was depleted and subsequently diagnosed with Chronic Fatigue Syndrome. It was only when my husband suggested trying for another baby, that I realised something had to change. I couldn't do this anymore and second time around would have to be different. I would have to learn to prioritise some of my own basic needs and I was going to explore how I could give myself a better chance at birthing.

I strongly believed, that if I could emerge from birth feeling physically and mentally stronger, this would provide me with a solid foundation from which to enter the next stage of motherhood, and embrace the slightly scary prospect of parenting not just one but two children!

This was really the turning point for me. For the first time, I actually began to realise that taking care of my own needs first and foremost was the most selfless thing to do. If I felt happier, calmer, more energised, then I would be a better mother as a result and have greater capacity to be there for my children in the way I wished to be.

My second birth was a very different experience and I am eternally grateful to HypnoBirthing for this. After completing the course and putting in a lot of home practice, I decided I would birth my second baby at home. The room was dimly lit by candlelight and soft music played in the background. Whilst I relaxed in the warmth of the birth pool, focused on my breathing and used positive visualisations, my husband Michael guided me through the birth using HypnoBirthing scripts, deepening techniques and prompts. Our midwives were tremendously supportive and simply sat back and observed whilst my husband and I gently and respectfully brought our son into the world. No pain, no fear, no manipulation, no forced pushing. All it took was a few gentle breaths to bring my baby safely and calmly into my husband's arms. Our HypnoBirth was truly a family event, and my daughter Eloise joined us to welcome Oscar into the world. When the birth was over I felt elated, alert and completely energised. I wanted to do it all over again, right there and then. Oscar scored top marks on the APGAR score, and fed and slept beautifully in the weeks to follow.

I knew then and there that I had to teach this method of birth preparation to other women. It changed my life, the way I viewed myself, the way I could mother, and led to a lifelong career advocating for women and children's mental and emotional wellbeing. I became a HypnoBirthing Instructor, supported and witnessed so many wonderful couples bring their babies calmly into the world, and subsequently launched Bloomii, a membership platform and loving community, that helps women grow mental resilience, emotional intelligence and build a daily habit of self care that lasts.

Ultimately, I believe we all have seeds of possibility within us, but in a busy world where our lives are so often led by the needs of others, we sometimes forget or find it hard to take care of ourselves in the way we deserve. If I was to give one piece of advice to any new mother it would absolutely be to never stop taking care of or loving yourself.

ROLE

Space to breathe
fill my lungs
close my eyes
empty arms
no touch but mine
forget my role
and find myself
slowly letting go
though it's true
I do miss you
I need time to be
a mama to no one
in this moment
but me

Holly Ruskin

SLEEP

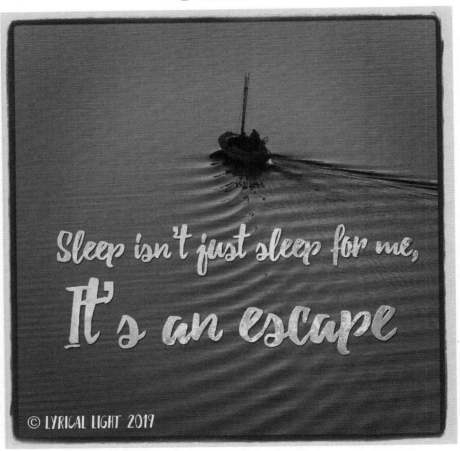

Sleep isn't just sleep for me, It's an escape

© LYRICAL LIGHT 2019

GEMMA

Rewrite The Fairytale

I t's a well known fact the mothers in fairytale stories don't come across too well. As little girls we listen to those stories of the woman who lived in a shoe, well she didn't know what to do? Jack's mum had to sell their only source of income, Mother Gothel locked her daughter in a tower and don't get me started on the warped views of step mums we grew up listening to. And even with there not being many positive stories of motherhood in our childhood stories, there are millions of children pushing toy buggies around, changing their babies nappies and dressing them in beautiful clothes. I can only think it's because being a mummy is amazing. Motherhood isn't always so.

I always knew I wanted to be a Mum. I love children and I was that cool auntie that would happily sit at the kids table. I was able to make up fun games to play, I bought the best presents and would be pleased to babysit whenever I was needed. I actually enjoy the company of children and get so much joy from seeing their joy too.

Now here comes the but.

But, motherhood is a total different kettle of chips. When you go to your new mum classes, they give you the lowdown on when to go to the hospital and they give you "that" importance of breast feeding chat. But nowhere does anyone tell you that if you make your bed and have a shower every morning you will feel like you can brace the day. They don't tell you that you need to write lists for everything because you will instantly forget what you needed in Tesco by the time you leave the house. Which, by the way, will take hours because you need to take a bag the size of a suitcase out with you everywhere!

This is where support comes in. A safe place to ask the questions you feel are silly or that you "should know". I feel so thankful that I have my mum and sister. I would happily send them a poo picture and ask if it looked normal? Which was usually yes. I was able to ask if it's normal to cry at pretty much everything some days, which was always "yes". And yet as much as they are amazing, I started to find myself making too much conversation with the checkout girl at Tesco because I hadn't had any adult interaction that day.

This is why, I believe, as much as it gets a bad rep sometimes, social media is so important. There are so many mums now sharing these moments in motherhood, which previously would feel like you were experiencing alone. I truly believe the greatest medicine for maternal mental health is knowing you are not alone. You are not alone in feeling lonely and suffocated at the same time, You are not alone in feeling grateful for your new life but also miss your old one. You are not alone in feeling joy and fear all at the same time. You are just not alone! There is nothing better than someone who has been there, done it, worn the milk stained T-shirt, saying

"I've been there, felt that, worn the same milk stained T-shirt"

Motherhood may not be the stuff of fairytales, but being a mummy is certainly the greatest story of them all.

LEAVE

They called it leave
but it was staying
staying with her
by her side instead
earning my living
by keeping her alive
never knowing when
my break would come
cold coffee
stale bread
no desk but a bed
to lie down
watch her
listen to her breathing
catch my breath
before doing it all
over and over and over
again
even less money
for infinite work
but if only I'd known
a smile
her laugh
little human happiness
my year end bonus

Holly Ruskin

FOREVER

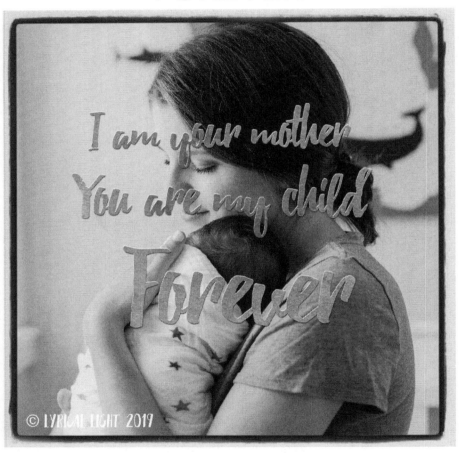

CERI

Feeling Like Myself Again

After being diagnosed with severe Postnatal Depression after the birth of my daughter Lucy, a tough road lay ahead for me and everybody who cared about me.

It had taken a lot of courage to go to the doctors but I knew I really wasn't feeling right and I couldn't go on hoping it would just sort itself out. It was hard to admit to myself that I needed help because to me I felt like I was too inadequate and weak to do so.

What I considered to be weakness, was in fact a real illness and it took a lot of time for me to see that and get over the guilt. No way would anybody choose to feel the terrible emotions I felt for over a year after Lucy's birth.

I knew motherhood was going to be hard but my experiences of early motherhood were in fact terrifying. That is the only way I can describe the confusion I felt. Everything to do with looking after Lucy overwhelmed me and I felt sheer panic from morning till night. I hardly slept (I got 2-3 hours for the first few weeks) and when I had a chance to sleep, I couldn't. My mind wouldn't slow down and the lack of sleep exacerbated my anxiety, panic and fear further. I experienced bad panic attacks for what seemed like no reason and I found looking after Lucy really surreal. She didn't feel like mine and my anxiety made me feel like there was no bond between us at all. I found taking her out in public really hard because I felt like the biggest fraud inside and I was worried people could see it. I dreaded being asked if I was enjoying being a mum because the answer was no, I really wasn't and it ate me up inside.

As you can imagine, this made me feel extremely low, I thought that I had made a huge mistake and that I didn't love Lucy. I felt I should never have become a mum and that I wasn't fit for the job. I was so scared of looking after Lucy that I never wanted to be on my own with her. When I tried to look after her alone I ended up having huge panic attacks and I felt like I was spiralling out of control.

No matter how positive I tried to be or how many pep talks my husband and I had, my feelings of panic and terror would always return. I remember Paul asking me where had his 'strong wife' gone and I honestly didn't know. I was convinced she would never return.

The guilt that comes with feeling like I did was massive and so another layer of misery was added to my woes. I thought I would never feel like me again and I couldn't see any future. I started to realise why people would want to end it all. I knew I couldn't go through with it though and so the living nightmare continued.

Lucy would cry first thing in the morning and I would wake up wishing that I hadn't. I can't tell you how scared I was to feel this way and how lonely I felt. I could have been in a room of hundreds of people and never have felt so alone in all my life.

My daughter would smile at me and all I felt was a huge, aching knot in my chest. I distinctly remember breast feeding her one day and throwing up whilst doing so. I also remember planning on running away and I went to the bus stop in my pyjamas and called my mum. Of course I knew I couldn't do it. It was definitely a cry for help. I really frightened my mum and husband that day and that's when my family knew that I needed to seek help.

When I look at the very few early photos of Lucy and me now, I find them really hard to look at. I can see in these photos that I wasn't really present, you can see it in my eyes. They were hiding sadness and conflict. I wish I could have those moments back and rewrite them because I do feel robbed of any happy memories of those early days.

Unfortunately, I also suffered from a lesser known illness called Post Natal OCD. Only 2 % of new mothers are diagnosed with this. I experienced frightening, intrusive thoughts and concluded these meant I was a danger to my daughter. In fact, I couldn't have been more wrong and that's why these thoughts plagued me. The more I tried to push them out of my mind or reason with them, the more they persisted. If I hadn't have sought professional help I would have continued thinking I was the monster I thought I was. Intrusive thoughts amongst new mothers are quite common but these thoughts can come and go without any weight attached to them. I was quite the opposite and the thoughts became a huge obsession that I would torture myself with and they continued for a long time before intervention helped me understand them.

It took medication and therapy to get me on the long road to recovery. I am a very impatient person and I had to face the fact that it was going to take time, not weeks or months but almost a year before I felt like the "Ceri before Lucy" again.

My daughter has given me strength that I didn't know existed and I am so lucky to be her mummy. I learn from her every day and thank my lucky stars that she is in my life.

I would like to thank my husband, family and all my friends who were there for me when I couldn't be there for myself. They never gave up on me and therefore I never gave up on me either.

SEAM

The days weave us closer
and the nights draw us in
so that where you end and I begin
there is no seam, no line or edge
just a merging and a pulling tight

Holly Ruskin

VICTORIA

Shadows And Light

My little boy has just turned 4. He's beautiful, lively, bright-eyed, happy and the light of my life. I love him to the ends of the Earth; I really do.

It's very hard to write this though, because although it's true, I feel so uneasy and sad. I feel uneasy and sad because I am still recovering from my pregnancy, his birth and what happened afterwards. My experiences of being pregnant with him, having him and then battling postnatal mental illness traumatised me. Everyone says that you'll never be the same after having a baby. It's true; you won't. I expected to change, but I thought it would be in a positive way along with some huge challenges, granted.

Bringing up a child is bloody hard work right from the word go. You are thrown in (sometimes it feels quite literally!) and you are responsible for another human being in every way. It's tough for everyone. I don't want sympathy; but I do think the mental state in which I found myself made it harder than it would be for many people.

I think I have always struggled with my mental health, but I first remember struggling with anxiety and depression at primary school. It wasn't picked up in those days. I struggled with relationships with peers and experienced bullying. I fought my way through school, went to university (battling through that too) and went on to train as a teacher. I've always been child-orientated and being a teacher and a mother, are things I'd had as life goals. I became a teacher and loved my job, but after some difficult life events, which led to even worse anxiety and depression, I had to stop. I had lost the ability to look after myself and went back to live with my parents.

I muddled along for a couple of years and then met Daniel. He literally changed my life and has supported me from the day I met him. I moved in with him and 2 years later we were married.

Falling pregnant was not easy for us. After a year of trying, I fell pregnant but didn't realise that I was. This baby died very early on and a sadly unhelpful experience at our Early Pregnancy Unit (EPU) ended up with me miscarrying in the toilet of a supermarket and then being told I'd lost the baby in the waiting room in front of other patients. I struggled to move on from this, but just wanted to be pregnant again.

I went on a health kick and a year later, I found myself pregnant again. From the word go, I was permanently on the edge of fear and anxiety if not fully immersed in them. I would go to the toilet to check that I wasn't bleeding every hour or so, even at work. My community midwife was wonderful, but concerned that I couldn't see that this pregnancy might result in a live baby. I was convinced that my baby was going to die and that

149

it would be my fault. I was physically and mentally exhausted throughout my pregnancy, suffering from exacerbated asthma and 3 chest infections. I enjoyed some of it and I was excited, but I never once relaxed. I couldn't; I might have missed something telling me that something was wrong.

When I got far enough along, I was told that I could go to the Day Assessment Unit (DAU) if I experienced reduced movement from my baby. I don't know if my son was ever not moving enough or whether anxiety told me he wasn't. To be honest, I think it probably happened once in the whole pregnancy. Anxiety took over, though and during the second half of my second trimester and for the entirety of my third trimester, the fantastic DAU were lucky if I wasn't in twice a week. At least.

I was in a pretty bad state. One midwife mentioned that I might be suffering from anxiety and I agreed(!) but I told her that medication was not an option. It would kill my baby, surely. Nothing more was done, despite my son being fine every time I was monitored. I think DAUs should be monitored by mental health services; I have met many others who have done similar things to me and it was all fuelled by anxiety and, on the whole, these mothers have gone on to have PND and the likes.

Eventually, when attending the DAU for the second time that week, and 4 days overdue, I was admitted for an induction. I was kind-of relieved...

The maternity ward was busy and they were not particularly attentive. Anxiety began to grip me as my pessaries kept failing me. I was left without one for around 14 hours when, finally, the overly-assertive and patronising midwife believed me when I said the pessary had fallen out.

Eventually, after a failed drip and a weird epidural and no progress, I was told I'd be having a c-section. I really didn't care. I just wanted to have this baby, get out of hospital and to sleep. I felt that I was alright and that once my baby was born, all would be resolved. From the Friday evening until that Monday evening when my son was born, I'd say I'd got around an hour's sleep. 1 hour in 72 hours. This is bad for anyone, let alone someone heavily pregnant and clearly anxious. Nothing was done or suggested to me and the staff knew what was happening.

The best part of the whole experience was when my little boy was cut out of me! He was perfect and I loved him immediately, which considering everything that was beginning to happen to me, was so lucky. We decided on his name right there and then.

This was where things got weird for me; almost immediately after his birth. I wasn't allowed to hold him and to see him very much; apparently I was bleeding badly, but no one had told me. I was cross and wanted to see him and just to have him close to me.

Suddenly, something in my head told me that he was called Leo. It was a name we'd discussed, but hadn't chosen it. Every time I spoke to my husband, I was calling our baby Leo. He was so sleep-deprived and in shock that I think this passed him by! I felt fuzzy and weird and gently happy, but there was something wrong...

Back in our room, with a healthy baby, my body wouldn't let me sleep. I would 'drop off' for seconds and then suddenly jolt back awake. Repeatedly. I remember talking to my mother-in-law who was dreamily holding her first grandson and telling myself that his name was Leo. I felt disassociated and unable to understand what she was saying.

I couldn't breastfeed successfully to start with (but it's so hard for many people!) One midwife told me my breasts were the wrong shape to breastfeed. Another told me I was on the verge of suffocating my son with my breasts. From then on, I was convinced I was going to kill him, in some way or another, through my inability to do anything to help him or to mother him. I felt like a complete fraud and as the hours went by, I felt less and less able to do ANYTHING. I don't remember eating anything either.

I was pretty much ignored by the maternity staff until, after various negative and traumatising experiences, including a maintenance man and a midwife walking in on me stark naked trying to breastfeed; my son's foot going purple and having to literally force them to do anything about removing the identity band from his ankle that was causing it, and a midwife walking into our room, pointing at my husband and saying,
"He has to leave. Right now," after my husband had been told he could stay with me, we decided to leave. Staff had shouted at us, I was seriously confused, exhausted and anxiety-fuelled and we felt that the only way to move forward was to go home to sleep.

They said we had to stay, but we fought to be discharged then and there. As I left, the same 'pessary incident' midwife said, "Watch out for any mania or feeling like you're going crazy." I had no idea what this meant, but shows that she had a full understanding of what was happening to me. She did not expand upon this statement when asked; nor did she pass on the information to anyone and I was left to it apart from the usual midwife and health visitor visits.

At home, I still couldn't sleep, whether my son was sleeping or not. He slept all day and was awake all night, seemingly. Still no sleep. My mum and Dan tried desperately to get me to sleep, but I would either refuse and start doing things manically or go up to bed and wait for sleep that was never coming.

Next, I stopped eating. Everything was a blur. I felt like I wasn't in my own body. Everyone was coming to see us, talking and trying to involve me. I was there, but I wasn't. Every little thing my son did or any little mark or change in behaviour would mean the end for him in my increasingly poorly mind. My mind told me I was neglectful and his illness or death was just inevitable with me as his mother.

Then, my mind took this darker and further. After about a week of still no sleep, I started to have images of myself putting my hand over his mouth. I kept it quiet, but every time I went near to my son, I would have these awful thoughts. It developed into everything I touched being a weapon to hurt my son. I thought I was always on the verge of killing him. I went to the GP and said that I thought I was schizophrenic and that I'd turned into an axe murderer. I wouldn't let my son be near me in case I hurt him and because being near him increased the thoughts.

The GP's first question was,
"But you're not actually going to do anything, are you? We have to ask to protect the baby."
I said, "No!" but underneath I was thinking,
"Yes, I am evil and I'm going to just lose it one day and do it."

153

I was prescribed anti-depressants. As soon as I got the prescription, I took one, desperate for something to stop the thoughts and the feelings. Of course, nothing as simple as a pill would have done anything at that point.

Still, no sleep.

I started to think my beloved cats were evil and that I didn't love them anymore. I stayed in bed for most of the days and nights and my husband fed my son. I googled frantically, seeing that what I was experiencing was a symptom of postnatal depression. It didn't help. I was a special case that couldn't be cured. I would spend the rest of my days with my son feeling like I was going to kill him. The situation seemed hopeless and completely unnerving. I felt like I was in a hole that I could never get out of. I started to think that I'd ruined my life by having a baby.

Eventually, the local crisis team believed our claims that this was an emergency and came on the same day. The two main nurses were helpful and empathetic and told me that it would get better. I didn't believe them. They told me I wouldn't hurt my baby; it was just my very poorly mind. I didn't believe this either. This was my life now, I was sure. Daily visits were good and check ins, but I kept asking Dan and my mum if they were talking about me behind my back. I started to think that they wanted to take my baby away from me.

One random crisis team worker came and asked me if social services were involved. That set me on another obsession. The health visitors and midwives and social services were on to me. They knew I was an imposter mother who did not deserve this beautiful child. I also felt that my job at a school was at risk if they heard about what had happened to me.

I was given sleeping pills and I gradually managed to sleep for some of the nights. Things started to get better, but I would NOT let anyone leave me alone with my son. My mum moved in with us because Dan had to go back to work. I did have an inner determination to continue holding and breastfeeding my son, so I did more and more every day. The thoughts didn't decrease and I learnt unhealthy ways to 'manage' them, to the point that I wouldn't let one of my arms near my son so as to be sure I wouldn't put my hand over his mouth. Incrementally, things got better, but it was slow. 4 months in and I would allow myself to be alone with my boy; my mum moved out but was on hand 24/7. I hated every minute, though. When I was alone, I was even less capable of controlling my mind. Everything seemed pointless.

The more I parented on my own, the more I realised that I wasn't going to do anything to my son. I still had the thoughts and they were horrible, but, with a recovery team (referred from the crisis team) they became less distressing. My mind had been playing tricks on me.

Only after I was discharged from the recovery team was I given a diagnosis of Severe Puerperal Behavioural Disorder, but having researched the process, I'm sure that I had (and now live with) Obsessive Compulsive Disorder (OCD.) I don't have OCD in the most widely-known sense (with obsessive cleaning and things being in their place or in a certain order) but I am completely obsessive about other things that worry me. My mind took me off into strange and horrible places. My thoughts make me play gambling games now e.g. 'If you do this in this way, everything will be ok,' or 'Stay off the pavement lines and Mum and Dad won't die,' Although I know that it is not real, I'm still taken me to dark places I never knew existed before I had a baby. It's very often overwhelming.

I love my son, but I still feel like a hopeless mother, especially when I am on my own. I can't think of my son as a baby and feel completely happy. I'm scarred.

Throughout my experiences, I wanted to meet other people who'd struggled with their perinatal mental health. I felt an urge to not feel alone. My psychiatric nurse told me not to speak to others who'd experienced these things because I'd start thinking that I had symptoms that they had and make myself worse. She could not have been more wrong.

If you are experiencing these things please find a support group. Finding others who had experienced these things changed my little, insular, mental illness world. I joined and then became the project manager of an art therapy group for mothers with PND and other perinatal mental illnesses. Meeting other mothers who 'just get it' helped immeasurably; I no longer felt completely alone, although I've still yet to meet anyone who has had these obsessive, intrusive thoughts about hurting their baby or child. I'd love to meet somebody who had them and is comfortable enough to talk about it. It's a taboo.

People don't talk about it (for seemingly obvious reasons, I guess.) Most people's reactions put me off. One health visitor (not on duty,) on me telling her what had happened and how I wanted to talk about it to help myself and others, said,
"Oh well, at least you're just talking about it and not actually acting on it, I guess."
Professionals working with new mothers need more training!

We're not immediate threats to our children; we're people who are ill. Yes, things can escalate, but in the majority of cases, if mothers and fathers are educated in their pregnancies and get the required help, things can be prevented and people recover.

I was going along, improving and feeling as comfortable as could be in my new normal. I started to get physically healthier and this improved my mental health too. I wanted another baby and, in October 2019, we were lucky enough to find out that I was pregnant, due in July, 2020. It had taken a lot of courage to make the decision to try for another baby because of my PND etc. However, finding out about our baby was a joyous moment. We were also coming to terms with the fact that our son most likely has Autistic Spectrum Disorder (ASD) and that, quite possibly, will need support as he goes to school and in his future life.

Then, in January, 2020, I had a late, missed miscarriage. My 12 weeks scan had been fine, but something, we don't know what, had happened. I had to fight to be listened to and scanned because I knew something was wrong. I went into labour naturally and gave birth to my poor, dead third baby, a sibling for my lovely boy and the completion to our family.

We asked for a post-mortem but we didn't feel able to find out the gender of our child or the strength to give them the funeral they deserved. I wish we had now, but at the time, it was unthinkable to us both.

In the midst of the global pandemic, shielding as an extremely vulnerable person, we found out that I have a duplication in one of my genes that I had passed on to my poor, sweet baby.

It hadn't caused the miscarriage, but it was likely to have been passed on to my son and that it's very possibly the cause of the probable ASD and other potential difficulties my son might have. My guilt continues and has been compounded by this. I am unlikely to have another baby and I've had to give up the work I was doing due to worsening mental and physical health and because of this pandemic.

I'd love to say that this is a story of hope. There is hope in some parts of my story. I no longer have specific thoughts of hurting my son and our relationship is very strong, but I'm the shell of who I was. I worry about everything. I don't enjoy a lot of the time that I spend with my son because I am plagued by the thought that I am failing him. It's probably the illness again, but it's something I can't see a way out of currently.

Things will improve, I am sure, but becoming a mother has shaped the last four years in a way I never thought it could. I am strong to have survived this, but I feel weak and lacking in any resilience after everything that has happened since 2016.

And this is what I find the hardest about my perinatal mental illness: the contradictions in the feelings I had/have. I love my son and I want the best for him, but the feelings and thoughts I had/have make time with him guilt-ridden and not as playful or as fun as I'd want them to be.

It's made me a shadow of a person and I'm still working my way out of this.

LETTER

You are the love letter
we wrote to ourselves
the only one
that won't fade over time
but in years to come
our words on your page
will grow as you do
even brighter

Holly Ruskin

MELISSA

The Power Of Music

I guess I've battled with depression for as long as I can remember. I'll go back to high school when I was maybe 12 or 13 and my parents split. My Dad moved out & that shattered me. I didn't get along with mum so well & my brother hated me. I was always in trouble though I could never work out what I was doing wrong.

Finally one day I guess my mum gave up and told my dad to come get me. I was to stay with him for a little while. About a week later she came over to talk and told me I had to choose which parent I was to live with. I chose my dad. She told me to come get my stuff on the weekend. We turned up on Saturday with boxes ready to pack up my room only to find she had already done it and it was all out on the porch. I didn't speak to her for a long time after that.

I met a guy when I was 15 who was a bad boy. I thought I loved him but he turned violent and I needed intervention to get him to leave me alone.

The next guy I met is the one who ruined me. I was already low and depressed and had no self confidence. He knew what he was doing. I fell hard for him.

The next 12 months were the worst in my life. I was at the point of being ready to reach out for help and the only person I felt comfortable enough going to was my cousin. I idolised him. We had a close relationship and he got me. I knew he would help me. Then we got the phone call that he had committed suicide. I was so lost and didn't know what to do. I also couldn't understand why I had such an intense anger. I stopped eating and caring.

My Lowest weight was about 42 kgs. I was in a bad way. I went to my doctor for a different issue but lucky for me he picked up what was going on. He prescribed anti depressants and told me this was my one and only chance. If I go back to him like that then he will put me in hospital. So I tried working my way back up the long and winding slope. My boyfriend just made things more difficult. He didn't like that he was losing control over me. I could write nearly a whole book on what that relationship was like but let's just say I finally reached my limit and managed to escape.

Fast forward a few years. It was time to really get my life on track and find work experience to get a job. I met my now husband. We were together for close to 2 years when I fell pregnant with our daughter. I was terrified but happy & healthy. She came 2 weeks early and all was good.

She took a bit of getting used to. The lack of sleep and being isolated at home (I didn't have friends because of my trust issues) caused depression to flare up again. Loneliness, frustration, anger.....yeah the anger is still there and I couldn't work out what I was so angry about. Mum was back in the picture and a massive support. Dad was and always had been there. My husband was brilliant. His family, however are not my biggest fans, but they didn't really cause any problems.

I just couldn't explain the anger I felt.

I went back to the doctor and was prescribed more anti depressants and this time a referral to a psychologist.
The psychologist is the man who saved me again and again over the next few years. I repeatedly went back to see him whenever things got bad.

As it turns out my constant anger was aimed at my cousin who committed suicide. He left when I needed him, I needed him to save me but he left.
I struggled constantly with complicated thoughts; how could I be angry at him? He had his own issues. It's not right that I feel anger towards him. I'm being selfish. That's just awful!
Well it just is what it is. We all have our feelings even if they don't make sense to us.

I'm now married, my daughter is 5, I have a part time job, a mortgage and my life is great. Time for child number 2.

That was a hard pregnancy with lots of pain and the lack of ability to physically do much. I packed the weight on and depression creept back in which wasn't helped by massive family arguments which caused lots of hurt feeing and emotional distance. Sadly it broke the relationship I had with my mum.

The baby was breach and that meant I had to have a c-section, but all went well with the birth and everyone was happy and healthy. I brought my beautiful baby home and all is good but I couldn't figure out why I was so sad and frustrated.

I remember looking at my son crying in his cot and having this intense urge to get in my car and drive away. I felt that I couldn't be left alone wtih the children, I was too messed up. I felt I just couldn't do it and I wanted out.

But then I really looked at my baby boy, my 5 year old princess and my ever-supportive husband and thought I was the worst person in the world! I knew I loved them all so much, so why did I want to leave? I was so tired of this cycle.

I went back to the psychologist, that man is a miracle worker. That was a hard slog back this time but here I am.

Fast forward to today. My son is now starting kindergarten and I'm so proud of him. I got a job during school hours and everyone's happy again.

After some bullying at my job I started my own little side business making embroidery and heat press items, and it's getting quite busy. I signed my daughter up for guitar lessons. and became friends with her teacher. He convinced me to move my business into the back of his guitar shop.

I spoke with my family and said it's now time to put me first a little bit. My kids are now 14 and 10. I'm ready to put me first and see what I can do with this business. Everything was going

163

RACHEL MASON

beautifully.

Covid hit! It hurt our business. So we made changes and ended up combining our businesses. So in the one shop we sell all things music related, do music lessons and all things heat press and embroidery related. I took a giant leap and started learning to play guitar and drums and it was the best thing I have ever done. My depression still rears up every now and then but it's nowhere near as bad and I am able to tell when I start to spiral and I reach out. I have an amazing support system with my family and friends. I am a big believer in using music to help your mood, whether you're playing it or listening to it. I always have music on now.

I am always happy to share my story. Especially if it's going to help someone else. Those dark times can be very confusing.

ACKNOWLEDGEMENTS

Writing a book is harder than I thought and more rewarding than I could have ever imagined. None of this would have been possible without my darling husband, Tom. He is my greatest supporter, sounding board, gives the best hugs and makes the perfect cup of tea. Tom has stood by me during every struggle and all my successes. Without his love and unswerving support I would not have made it through the darkest days of my postnatal depression.

I also want to thank:

Every single one of the brave and amazing parents who sent me their very personal story to be included in this book. Without you there would be no book. You are all incredible and your stories will help so many people.

Holly Ruskin for the beautiful poetry and for sharing her talents with me for this book.

Lisa Timms for the gorgeous cover illustration.

Luke for the fantastic graphic design and endless patience.

Olivia Siegl for the lovely foreword, letter of light and for being the most honest and kind-hearted woman I've had the pleasure to know. Olivia's book Bonkers got me through some tough times with my own postnatal depression and for that I'll be forever grateful.

My wonderful parents for their endless love and support of every crazy idea I've ever had. Dad for telling me I can't and Mum for telling me I can.

My beautiful children, Layla and Elias. The lights of my life and my greatest ever achievement.

My dear friends Caroline and Emma who are the best mum and musical theatre friends a girl could wish for. I love that our children are growing up together and adore each other as much as I adore you.

My sister Rosie and brother in law Jon for their constant love, support and vegan cake.

My bestie Abi for always loving me no matter what life throws at us.

Faye and all the awesome women at Freelance Mum who support and inspire me every single day. You are my tribe and I can't imagine my life without you.

Kirsty for the wonderful photography and laughter.

Maria at Mothers For Mothers for her bravery and kindnessss.

Annie and the team at PANDAS for everything.

Mummy Social for all the support.

Rosey at PND and Me for her advice.

Anna at Motherdom Magazine for championing Lyrical Light and for introducing me to Lisa and Luke without whom the cover of this book wouldn't be nearly as awesome.

Lizzie and Xav at Bare Wall Studios for making all the Lyrical Light tracks and being generally wonderful.

Helen at Bloomii for the Hypnobirthing training and for giving such calm and balanced advice.

Laura Rawlings at BBC Radio Bristol for championing Lyrical Light and this book.

My wonderful church family at Clevedon Baptist Church for your love and prayers, especially Luke, Jo and Gemma and to Kristen for making the most delicious banofee pie to cheer me up.

I want to thank EVERYONE who ever said anything positive to me or taught me something. I heard it all, and it meant something.

The entire staff of St Michael's Hospital Maternity Department in Bristol for taking such good care of my two babies, Tom, Rosie and me during two long and difficult births.

I want to thank God most of all, because without God I wouldn't be able to do any of this.

ABOUT THE AUTHOR

Rachel Mason

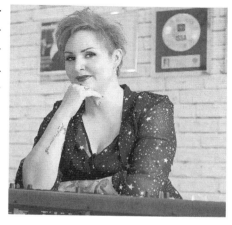

Rachel Mason is a multi-award-winning singer, songwriter, author, tv music judge and philanthropist who is based in North Somerset in the United Kingdom.

A survivor of postnatal depression and Patron for Vine Counselling Services, Rachel writes about her experiences for publications including Motherdom Magazine, Guilty Mother's Club, Authentic, Mental Movement and Authority Magazine. She is an ambassador for maternal mental health and gives her time to run Lyrical Light songwriting workshops for those with maternal mental health issues, creating personalised songs to aid in their recovery. For this groundbreaking work Rachel has been hailed "an inspiration" by Prince Harry.

Rachel is the only musician to have been crowned Freelancer of the Year and runs an artist management business, record label and multiple choirs alongside her vocal coaching business, charity work and raising her two young children.

ABOUT THE AUTHOR

Lisa Timms

Lisa lives in Hertfordshire with her Husband and two boys, Luca and Robin. She reconnected with her artistic roots after recognising the need for a creative outlet and escape for busy mums with her First Mummies' Club evening workshops, which ran for several years at various venues in Herts.

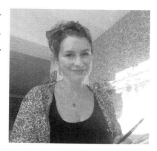

Lisa has most recently been providing illustrations to accompany parents' stories surrounding maternal mental health in Motherdom magazine for the last year. It's a role that has encouraged her to consider the different ways we can communicate ideas and emotions that are sometimes tricky to verbalise, aiming to depict the joy of humour in situations that parenthood can often present us with.

Lisa is delighted to contribute her illustrations to a book which acknowledges the mental health struggles parents face and celebrate the importance of Mothers and Fathers sharing their experiences with the world.

@firstmummiesclub

ABOUT THE AUTHOR

Holly Ruskin

Holly studied English Literature and Film
at University of Exeter, graduating in 2005
and embarking on a career in education.
She finished her MA in Film and Television
at University of Bristol in 2018 and now
lectures in Film and Media, specialising in
motherhood, gender and feminist theory.

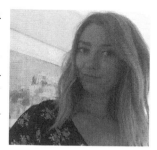

She has been a writer all her life but started exploring the poetic
form after the birth of her daughter in 2019. After being diagnosed with birth trauma and postnatal depression, she began
writing poems about her experiences and sharing them online
as @mother.in.motion.

Having edited screenplays, written short stories and academic
essays, it is writing poems about motherhood that has brought
her the most creative joy. Snatching time in between feeding,
napping and playing with her daughter - often before the rest
of the world wakes up - her collection has slowly evolved into
something that she hopes any mother or parent can connect
with.

She is the co-founder and editor of the online poetry journal
'blood moon poetry', an inclusive and welcoming place for fe-
male poets to submit their work for publication. She is also
working with other creative women on a range of collaborative

projects.

Holly lives in Bristol, UK.

PRAISE FOR AUTHOR

A beautifully written book. The honesty of these brave parents will provide invaluable support for others who may be suffering in silence.

- EMMA HARVEY, NHS MIDWIFE

Postnatal depresion affects so many parents and it can be hard to talk about. That is why 'Not the Only One' is a huge benefit to so many parents to help them realise they are not alone and that there is a way forward.

- CHERYL LEE-WHITE, BEST-SELLING AUTHOR AND POET

Rachel gives a voice to those of us who have suffered in silence. Showing that depression, far from being a sign of failure is an invitation to know ourselves more deeply and turn towards our networks of support, being nurtured by the village as we nurture our child. It is our system crying out for what we know deep down that we need. Listen to these stories and know you are not alone.

- NINA BAMBREY, AUTHOR OF SPIRITED

The real-life stories in this book are heartwarmingly reassuring. When we start our journey to becoming parents we have no idea what is truly ahead of us. This beautifully written book brings together the many different paths that parents have travelled and the challenges that they have faced. These stories are proof that we're not travelling alone. That we have more courage than we think. And asking for help has nothing to do with our ability to parent.

By writing this book, Rachel has not only shone a light on the struggles that so many parents face but also the abundance of love that parents have for their children.

- MARIA A NEWMAN, BLOGGER AND CREATOR OF MUMMY ON A BREAK PODCAST

Perinatal Mental Health has come a long way in recent years and this book will cement what all parents, campaigners and professionals have been fighting for to help and improve society.
This book demonstrates the power of voices of lived experiences in a time when very few are given the opportunity, and also to educate this generation and generations to come that it is ok to say you're not ok.
Not The Only One is a great resource and a book that I use to support parents in seeking the help they need.

- MARK WILLIAMS, AUTHOR OF DADDY BLUES AND TEDX TALKS KEYNOTE SPEAKER

Postnatal depression has had a huge impact on the lives of everyone in my family. With both our kids my wife experienced PND - most impactfully with our second child. My wife fell into a deep depression which led to suicidal thoughts and attempts.

Through all of this the overwhelming feeling was one of isolation. Whilst postnatal depression was discussed in medical circles it seems to be met with silence in social circles. We felt totally alone and even ashamed that this was happening to us. I vicious cocktail of guilt, loneliness, helplessness and fear only served to enhance the, already crippling, cloud of despair that had fallen.

As a man I'm this situation I felt the impact too. Juggling a career, newborn, my daughter (who is autistic) and my wife became almost impossible. My wife needed my support whilst I was also committed to my work. My family felt like it was crumbling around me and I felt lost. Again the silence in my peers made this a very lonely time. I felt like no one understood what was happening. I felt a failure - as though this was my fault. I felt helpless and hopeless.

The title of Rachel's book, Not the Only One, cuts right to the bone of what so many of us need to know. Countless millions experience PND, and finally people are speaking up and sharing their experiences to destigmatise the topic.

But even more it's a support! Being able to dip in and out is such a comfort. Knowing we're far from alone in this battle is such a relief. These shared experiences feel like warm hugs lifting from the pages.

I recommend this book to anyone who's starting their parenthood journey, already a parent, and especially to anyone experiencing the silent killer that is postnatal depression. You're not alone, far from it; you're actually in fine company! Not the Only One will lift your spirits, give you comfort in even the darkest moments, and starts the massively overdue conversation that's sorely needed.

- DUNCAN CASBURN, CREATOR OF YOUTUBE'S PDA DAD UK

This is the book that all new parents should read.

- FAYE DICKER, FREELANCE MUM

Honest, raw and relatable. A much-needed collection of of real life parenthood experiences and the struggles so many face.

- ROSEY ADAMS, PND AND ME

These stories will bring comfort to those that have been there and illumination to to those who haven't.

- KATIE SILVERTHORNE, AUTHOR

Rachel Mason's exploration of the effects of PND on a wide variety of parents is a fascinating insight into a condition that is so often not discussed, not least by parents themselves. By turns inspiring and uplifting, as well as deeply moving, this book is a much needed window into the condition, and one that not only sheds light on PND, but also offers hope to those who might be struggling to make sense of themselves, their relationships and the new additions to their lives in the aftermath of a birth. A must read for parents at all stages!

- FAY KEENAN, BEST-SELLING AUTHOR

Moving, honest and heartwarming. I finally feel like someone understands what I went through after I had my baby and cares about me.

- AARNA PATEL, MOTHER

Not The Only One is perfectly titled. When you read this book you'll know you're not alone. So many parents face mental health challenges and feel ashamed, isolated, or too scared to ask for help. I know - I was one of those. Rachel has brought together mums and dads to break down the stigma of maternal and paternal mental ill-health.

- ANNA CEESAY, FOUNDING EDITOR OF MOTHERDOM, THE UK'S FIRST MEDIA PLATFORM DEDICATED TO MATERNAL MENTAL HEALTH AND WELLBEING

Reading this is like having a community of lived experience around you. If you've ever wondered about the reality of PND, here are the voices who made it out the other side.

- ANGIE BELCHER, STAND UP COMEDIAN AND WRITER

Not The Only One offers any parent fantastic support in their mental health struggles and shows us all we really aren't alone.

- MUMMY SOCIAL

Rachel perfectly captures the confusion of emotions and the reality of motherhood for men and women suffering from loneliness, anxiety and depression during the pregnancy or after their baby has been born.
She does the unthinkable by bringing beauty and grace to such a difficult subject. The diverse experiences, the stories and the poetry ensure that there is something in this collection for everyone.
The gift of this book is truly letting mums and dads know that they are "Not the Only One"

- MARIA VINER, CHIEF EXECUTIVE OFFICER MOTHERS FOR MOTHERS

Not the Only One is a powerful and reassuring read for mums, Dads, grandparents and staff who are either affected by or supporting someone with postnatal depression of other forms of perinatal mental health conditions. With some very honest and heartfelt accounts and poems from mums and dads who have experienced this first hand, the book enables you really put yourself into their shoes to understand their feelings and experiences. I would thoroughly recommend this to anyone who needs support-it not only provides reassurance that you are definitely Not the Only One but also some insight and positivity into recovery.

- CLAIRE BULLOCK, SOUTH WEST PERINATAL AND INFANT MENTAL HEALTH PROGRAMME MANAGER FOR NHS ENGLAND

Rachel shares honest stories from the community showing that postnatal depression does not discriminate. It offers hope by passing on the knowledge that this is not something that needs to be hidden, but that this very place of pain can be something that brings people together and that a stigma can be transformed by simply realising you are not alone.

- SARAH LUGG, CREATOR OF REAL HONEST MOTHER

These stories are straight from the heart - told openly and honestly. What it is like to be in the midst of an incredibly dark time but also sharing the recovery. There is light and hope - a powerful anchor for anyone wondering 'is it just me?'

- LAURA RAWLINGS, BBC JOURNALIST AND CLINICAL HYPNOTHERAPIST

Printed in Great Britain
by Amazon

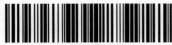
50115141R00118